VITALITY GUIDE TO ISOMETRIC EXERCISES FOR SCOLIOSIS

Strengthen Your Spine, Achieve Stability with Safe and Effective Isometric Training

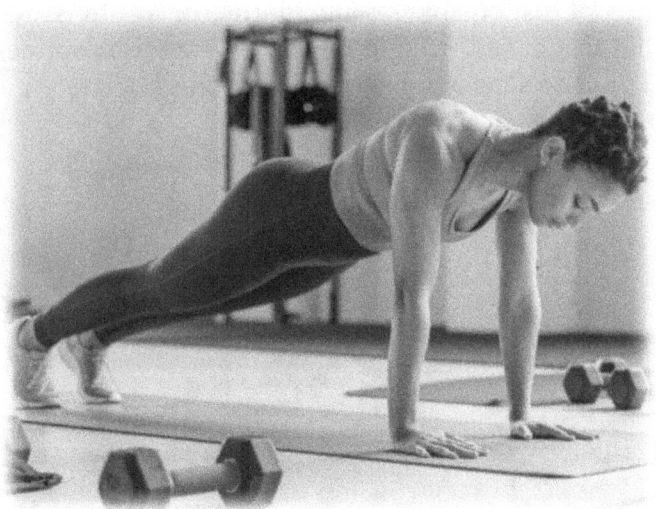

Caren Woods

Copyright © 2024 Caren Woods

All Rights Reserved

Disclaimer

Before beginning any exercise program, including the exercises described in this book, it is important to consult with your healthcare provider to ensure the activities are appropriate for your individual health and fitness level. The exercises and information provided in this book are for educational purposes only and should not be used as a substitute for professional medical advice, diagnosis, or treatment. The author and publisher are not responsible for any injuries or health issues that may result from following the exercise routines or suggestions provided in this book.

Table of Contents

VITALITY GUIDE TO ISOMETRIC EXERCISES FOR SCOLIOSIS i

Table of Contents iii

Introduction: Why This Book and How to Use It 1

Chapter 1: Understanding Isometric Exercises for Scoliosis 3

    What Are Isometric Exercises? 4

    Benefits of Isometric Exercises for Scoliosis 8

    How Isometric Exercises Fit into Scoliosis Management 13

Chapter 2: Addressing Misconceptions About Isometric Exercises...17

    Understanding the Limitations of Exercises Alone..22

    The Importance of Professional Guidance..27

Chapter 3: Core Isometric Exercises 32

    Plank Variations for Core Stability 33

    Side Planks for Oblique Strength................39

    Modified Planks for Beginners...................45

Chapter 4: Upper Body Isometric Exercises...52

    Wall Push-Ups for Shoulder Strength 53

    Isometric Rows for Back Muscles 59

Resistance Band Holds for Upper Body Balance 66

Chapter 5: Lower Body Isometric Exercises ... 74

Wall Sits for Leg Strength 75

Glute Bridges for Hip Stability 82

Isometric Lunges for Muscle Imbalance Correction 89

Chapter 6: Postural and Spine-Supportive Isometric Exercises 97

Wall Angels for Improved Posture 99

Scapular Squeezes for Shoulder Blade Strength 106

Pelvic Tilts for Lower Back Support 113

Chapter 7: Isometric Exercises for Daily Activities 120

Chair Sits for Office Workouts 122

Isometric Walking Drills for Improved Balance 129

Core Engagement While Standing 136

Chapter 8: Safety and Progression in Isometric Exercises 144

Starting with Short Holds and Gradual Increases 146

Recognizing and Avoiding Painful Movements 152

Tracking Progress for Motivation 159

Chapter 9: Nutrition to Support Scoliosis Management 166

Bone-Strengthening Nutrients: Calcium and Vitamin D 167

Muscle-Supportive Nutrients: Protein, Magnesium, and Potassium 172

Importance of Hydration and Balanced Meals 179

Chapter 10: Putting It All Together 186

Building a Weekly Isometric Exercise Plan 187

Combining Isometric Workouts with Other Treatments 192

Sustaining Long-Term Results 197

Conclusion 203

Introduction: Why This Book and How to Use It

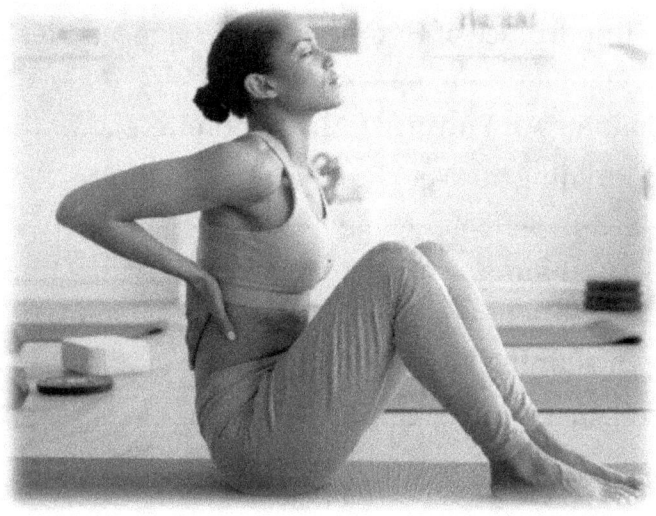

Isometric exercises involve muscle engagement without movement, offering stability and strength. For individuals with scoliosis, these exercises can improve posture, reduce discomfort, and enhance daily function. This guide empowers readers to safely integrate isometric techniques into their routines, fostering alignment and confidence through targeted, practical strategies for spinal health.

Chapter 1: Understanding Isometric Exercises for Scoliosis

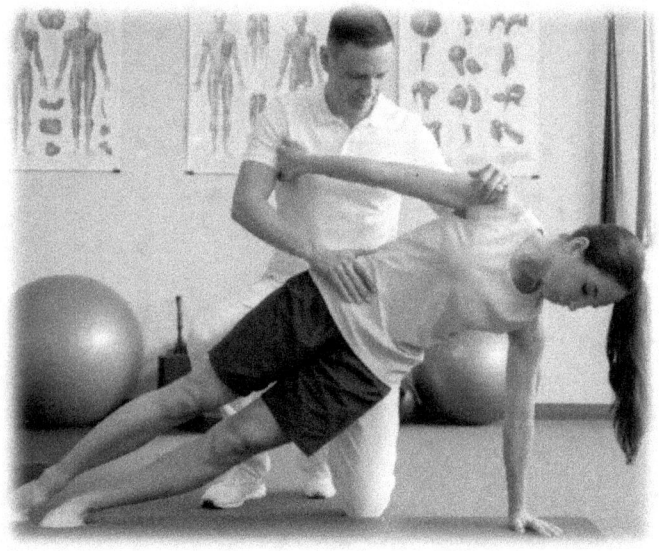

Isometric exercises are movements where muscles contract without visibly changing length, providing strength and stability without joint motion. These exercises are especially valuable for individuals with scoliosis, as they build core stability and improve posture without exacerbating spinal curvature. Understanding their mechanics can empower you to manage scoliosis more effectively.

What Are Isometric Exercises?

At their heart, isometric exercises are all about holding a position that engages specific muscle groups. Imagine holding a plank position or pressing your palms together with force—your muscles are working hard, but there's no noticeable movement. This static contraction builds endurance and strength in a way that's gentler on your joints than dynamic exercises.

For scoliosis, the lack of movement is key. Dynamic exercises, which involve repetitive motion, can sometimes place stress on uneven spinal curves. Isometric exercises, on the other hand, stabilize and strengthen the supporting muscles, helping your body maintain better alignment.

Why They Matter for Scoliosis

Scoliosis involves a sideways curve of the spine, often accompanied by muscle imbalances. Some muscles may be overworked and tight, while others are weak and underused. Isometric exercises help address these imbalances. When you perform an isometric hold, you're not just strengthening muscles; you're also training them to support your spine more evenly.

These exercises are safe and adaptable. You can adjust the intensity to suit your strength level and gradually increase the challenge as you become more comfortable. This makes them an ideal option for people with varying degrees of scoliosis.

Examples of Isometric Exercises

Here are a few examples to help you visualize what isometric exercises look like:

1. Wall Sits

Sit with your back against a wall as if you're in an invisible chair. Hold this position for 15-30 seconds, focusing on engaging your core and keeping your spine straight.

2. Plank Holds

Support your body on your forearms and toes, keeping your back flat and your core engaged. Start with 10-20 seconds and increase gradually.

3. Side Plank Modifications

Lie on your side and lift your hips off the ground, supporting yourself on one forearm. This targets the oblique muscles, which are often imbalanced in scoliosis.

The Science Behind Isometric Training

When you hold a muscle contraction, blood flow to the area increases, delivering oxygen and nutrients while flushing out waste. This process strengthens the muscle fibers and improves endurance. Additionally, isometric exercises enhance proprioception—your body's awareness of its position—which is particularly helpful for correcting posture in scoliosis.

Practical Tips to Get Started

1. Start Small

Begin with shorter hold times, such as 10-15 seconds, and gradually increase as your strength improves.

2. Focus on Alignment

Pay attention to your posture during each exercise. Use a mirror or guidance from a physical therapist to ensure correct positioning.

3. Breathe

Avoid holding your breath while contracting your muscles. Breathe steadily to help maintain focus and relaxation.

4. Include Rest Periods

Allow your muscles time to recover between exercises to prevent fatigue or strain.

Strategic Suggestions

To incorporate isometric exercises into your scoliosis management plan, start with two to three sessions per week, focusing on exercises that target your core, back, and hips. Pair these with stretching to improve flexibility and release tight muscles. With consistency, you'll notice improved posture, strength, and confidence in managing your scoliosis.

Benefits of Isometric Exercises for Scoliosis

Isometric exercises offer a unique approach to managing scoliosis. Their focus on static muscle engagement promotes strength, stability, and alignment, making them particularly beneficial for individuals with spinal curvature. Understanding how these exercises contribute to physical well-being can help you build a more supportive and effective routine.

Improving Posture and Spinal Stability

One of the most noticeable benefits of isometric exercises is their ability to improve posture. With scoliosis, maintaining a balanced posture can be challenging due to uneven muscle tension around the spine. Isometric exercises directly address this issue by engaging the muscles responsible for supporting the spine, such as the core, back, and hip muscles.

For instance, holding a plank strengthens the deep abdominal muscles and the muscles along the spine. These muscles act as a natural brace, helping to counteract the pull of scoliosis and encouraging better alignment. Over time, this can lead to noticeable improvements in how you sit, stand, and move.

Building Symmetrical Strength

Scoliosis often creates muscle imbalances, where one side of the body is stronger or more developed than the other. Isometric exercises are an effective way to target these imbalances. Because you're holding a position rather than moving dynamically, you can focus on engaging weaker muscles without overcompensating with stronger ones.

Take the side plank, for example. This exercise specifically targets the obliques and lateral stabilizers, which are often asymmetrical in individuals with scoliosis. When you perform this exercise on both sides, you can gradually build more symmetrical strength, improving overall balance and coordination.

Reducing Pain and Discomfort

Chronic pain is a common issue for people with scoliosis, often caused by muscle tension and strain. Isometric exercises can help alleviate this pain by promoting muscle relaxation and improving circulation. When muscles contract and hold during an isometric exercise, they release tension and become more resilient over time.

Additionally, the increased blood flow during isometric holds delivers oxygen and nutrients to the muscles, aiding in recovery and reducing inflammation. Exercises like the wall sit or bridge pose can relieve discomfort in the lower back and hips, common areas of tension for those with scoliosis.

Enhancing Core Strength

A strong core is essential for anyone with scoliosis, as it provides the foundation for a stable and supported spine. Isometric exercises are particularly effective for targeting the deep core muscles, including the transverse abdominis and multifidus, which play a crucial role in spinal stability.

The plank is a prime example of a core-strengthening isometric exercise. When you hold the plank position, you engage multiple muscle groups simultaneously, including the abdominals, back, shoulders, and legs. This integrated approach to core strengthening helps distribute forces evenly across the body, reducing stress on the spine.

Promoting Better Body Awareness

Isometric exercises also enhance body awareness, or proprioception. This is your ability to sense and control your body's position and movements. For individuals with scoliosis, improving proprioception is invaluable for correcting posture and maintaining alignment during daily activities.

When you practice isometric exercises, you're training your brain to recognize and adjust to better posture. For example, holding a wall sit teaches you to maintain a neutral spine and engage the correct muscles, which can translate to better posture throughout the day.

Safe and Accessible for All Levels

One of the greatest advantages of isometric exercises is their adaptability. They can be tailored to suit your fitness level and modified as you progress. No matter if you're new to exercise or more experienced, isometric holds can be adjusted to provide an appropriate level of challenge.

For example, beginners might start with modified planks on their knees, while more advanced individuals can incorporate weights or extend hold times for added intensity. This versatility makes isometric exercises a safe and effective option for managing scoliosis across all stages of life.

Strategic Suggestions

To get the most out of isometric exercises, focus on consistency and technique. Start with short holds and gradually increase duration as your strength improves. Use mirrors or guidance to ensure proper alignment, and pair these exercises with gentle stretching to maintain flexibility. With dedication, you'll see noticeable improvements in strength, posture, and comfort.

How Isometric Exercises Fit into Scoliosis Management

Isometric exercises are more than just a workout; they're a powerful tool for managing scoliosis. These exercises strengthen supporting muscles, improve spinal stability, and complement other treatments. When integrated thoughtfully into your routine, they can become a cornerstone of a holistic approach to scoliosis care.

Supporting a Comprehensive Management Plan

Scoliosis management often includes multiple strategies, such as physical therapy, bracing, or, in some cases, surgery. Isometric exercises fit seamlessly into this framework by targeting muscle imbalances and enhancing the spine's structural support. They provide a gentle, controlled method for improving muscle strength without risking further stress to the spine.

For example, if you're undergoing physical therapy, isometric exercises can reinforce the techniques you learn in your sessions. Exercises like the bridge pose or side plank can be performed at home to maintain progress between appointments.

Additionally, if you're wearing a brace, isometric exercises strengthen the muscles that the brace supports, creating a synergistic effect that improves alignment over time.

Addressing Muscle Imbalances

Scoliosis creates a unique set of challenges due to uneven muscle development. Some muscles may be overactive, pulling the spine further into its curve, while others may be underactive, providing little support. Isometric exercises are particularly effective at addressing these imbalances because they allow you to isolate and engage specific muscles.

Take the side plank, for example. Holding this position on the weaker side of your body can gradually strengthen underactive muscles, promoting better symmetry and reducing the strain on overworked areas.

Promoting Consistency and Longevity

One of the greatest strengths of isometric exercises is their simplicity and accessibility. You don't need fancy equipment or a gym membership to incorporate them into your routine. This makes it easier to stay consistent, which is critical for long-term scoliosis management.

For instance, you can perform a wall sit while watching TV or a plank during a short break in your day. These exercises are quick to perform but deliver long-lasting benefits, making them an excellent choice for busy lifestyles.

Preventing Progression

While isometric exercises cannot "cure" scoliosis, they play a vital role in preventing further progression of the curve. When you strengthen the muscles that support your spine, you can reduce the mechanical stress that contributes to worsening alignment.

This is particularly important for adolescents with idiopathic scoliosis, whose curves may still be developing. Regular isometric exercises can help slow progression and maintain better posture as their bodies grow.

Complementing Other Forms of Exercise

Isometric exercises work best when paired with other forms of physical activity, such as stretching, aerobic exercise, and dynamic strength training. Together, these activities create a balanced approach to scoliosis management that addresses flexibility, cardiovascular health, and overall muscle strength.

For example, you might combine isometric holds with yoga poses to improve flexibility or add light resistance training to build overall muscle endurance. The key is to create a routine that supports your individual needs and goals.

Adapting Exercises for Individual Needs

Scoliosis varies widely in severity and presentation, so it's important to tailor isometric exercises to your specific condition. Consulting with a physical therapist or healthcare professional can help you identify the best exercises for your unique spinal curve.

For example, if your scoliosis primarily affects your lumbar spine, you might focus on isometric exercises that target the lower back and hips. On the other hand, if your thoracic spine is more affected, exercises like wall presses or seated rows may be more beneficial.

Strategic Suggestions

To make isometric exercises a lasting part of your scoliosis management plan, schedule short sessions 3-4 times a week. Pair these exercises with activities that improve flexibility and cardiovascular health for a balanced approach. Stay mindful of your body's responses, and seek professional guidance to ensure your routine aligns with your needs.

Chapter 2: Addressing Misconceptions About Isometric Exercises

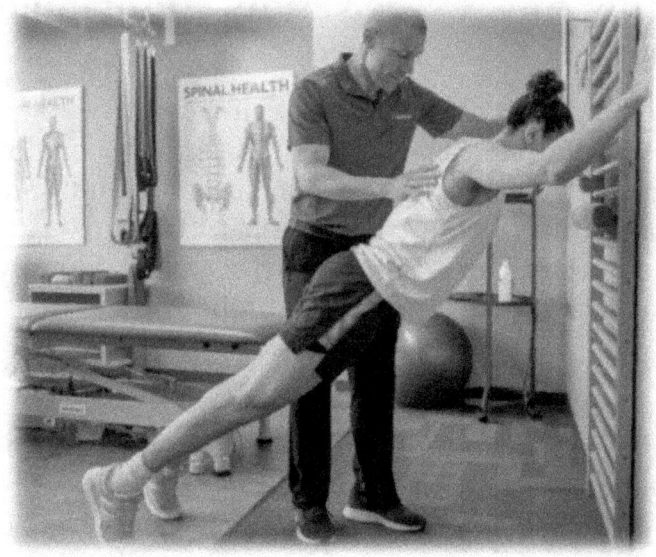

When it comes to isometric exercises for scoliosis, misinformation can create confusion and discourage progress. Many misconceptions exist about their effectiveness, safety, and role in scoliosis management. Addressing these myths and understanding the facts will empower you to make informed decisions and use these exercises to their fullest potential.

Common Myths and Realities

Myth 1: Isometric Exercises Can Cure Scoliosis

One of the most common misconceptions is that isometric exercises can completely reverse scoliosis. The truth is that while these exercises can significantly improve muscle strength, posture, and overall comfort, they cannot eliminate the spinal curvature.

Scoliosis is a structural condition, meaning it involves changes to the spine's shape and alignment. Isometric exercises are a management tool, not a cure. They work by strengthening the muscles that support your spine, which can reduce the progression of the curve and improve your quality of life. Think of them as a way to control the condition, not to erase it.

Myth 2: Isometric Exercises Are Unsafe for Scoliosis

Another misconception is that isometric exercises might be harmful or worsen the spinal curve. This is far from true when the exercises are done correctly. Isometric exercises involve static holds, which reduce the risk of strain or injury compared to dynamic exercises with repeated movements.

These exercises are gentle on the joints and can be tailored to your specific needs. For example, planks or wall sits can be modified to accommodate your comfort level while still providing the muscle engagement you need. If you focus on proper form and start with manageable hold times, isometric exercises are both safe and effective.

Myth 3: Only Children with Scoliosis Can Benefit

Scoliosis is often associated with adolescence, but the condition can affect individuals of any age. Many believe that adults with scoliosis won't see much benefit from isometric exercises, but this isn't the case.

While the goals may differ—adolescents might focus on preventing curve progression, while adults aim to manage pain and improve posture—both groups can benefit. For older adults, isometric exercises are particularly valuable as they're low-impact and easy to integrate into daily routines.

Myth 4: Isometric Exercises Are Too Simple to Be Effective

Because isometric exercises don't involve dynamic movement, some people underestimate their power. However, these exercises are highly effective for building muscle endurance, improving stability, and addressing imbalances, especially for conditions like scoliosis.

For example, holding a plank may seem simple, but it engages multiple muscle groups simultaneously, including your core, back, and shoulders. The lack of movement doesn't make these exercises less effective—it ensures controlled engagement, which is perfect for individuals with scoliosis.

Myth 5: You Need Expensive Equipment or a Gym

Many believe that effective exercise requires access to specialized equipment or a gym membership. Isometric exercises, however, are wonderfully accessible. You can perform them anywhere—at home, at work, or even outdoors—using nothing more than your body weight.

For example, a wall sit only requires a sturdy wall, and a plank can be done on any flat surface. This accessibility makes it easier to incorporate these exercises into your routine, ensuring consistency and long-term benefits.

The Realities of Isometric Exercises

Now that we've addressed the myths, let's focus on the facts. Isometric exercises are an essential part of scoliosis management because they:

1. **Strengthen Core and Supporting Muscles**

These exercises target the muscles that hold your spine in place, improving alignment and stability.

2. **Reduce Pain and Discomfort**

Isometric exercises releases muscle tension and promote blood flow, which help alleviate common pain associated with scoliosis.

3. **Improve Posture and Proprioception**

They teach your body to hold itself in better alignment, enhancing awareness and reducing strain during daily activities.

4. **Are Low-Impact and Adaptable**

They're safe for people of all ages and can be adjusted to match your fitness level.

Strategic Suggestions

To maximize the benefits of isometric exercises, focus on proper form, consistent practice, and realistic expectations. Recognize that these exercises are part of a broader scoliosis management plan. Partner with a professional to tailor a program to your needs, and let the truth about isometric exercises guide your path to better spinal health.

Understanding the Limitations of Exercises Alone

While exercises, including isometric ones, play a significant role in managing scoliosis, they are not a standalone solution. Understanding the scope and limitations of these exercises helps set realistic expectations and ensures you integrate them effectively into a broader scoliosis management plan.

What Exercises Can and Cannot Do

Exercises like planks, wall sits, and side holds target the muscles that support your spine, improving strength, balance, and stability. These benefits can enhance posture, reduce pain, and even slow the progression of scoliosis in some cases. However, it's crucial to remember that exercises cannot correct the structural changes in your spine caused by scoliosis.

Think of isometric exercises as a support system. They reinforce the muscles that hold your spine, making daily activities easier and more comfortable. But these exercises alone cannot reshape the spine's natural curve or fully address severe imbalances. For structural changes, other interventions, like bracing or surgery, might be necessary depending on the severity of your condition.

The Need for a Multifaceted Approach

Scoliosis management is most effective when it combines several strategies, tailored to the individual's needs. These strategies often include:

1. Physical Therapy

Guided sessions can complement isometric exercises, focusing on techniques like spinal mobilization and muscle activation.

2. Bracing

For growing children and adolescents, bracing helps prevent the curve from worsening.

3. Stretching and Flexibility Training

While isometric exercises strengthen muscles, stretching helps release tension in tight areas, balancing the effects of scoliosis.

4. Regular Medical Monitoring

X-rays and check-ups are crucial for tracking scoliosis progression, especially in younger individuals.

Isometric exercises should be seen as one piece of the puzzle rather than the entire picture. When combined with these other elements, they can make a significant impact on your overall quality of life.

Recognizing When Exercises Alone Are Not Enough

1. Rapid Curve Progression

For adolescents whose spines are still growing, scoliosis can progress quickly. In these cases, bracing or other interventions might be necessary.

2. Severe Pain or Discomfort

While isometric exercises can reduce pain, persistent or worsening pain may require additional treatment, such as physical therapy or medical intervention.

3. Breathing or Functional Limitations

In severe cases of scoliosis, the spinal curve can affect lung capacity or mobility, requiring more advanced care.

Being aware of these limitations doesn't diminish the value of isometric exercises. Instead, it highlights the importance of working with professionals to create a personalized management plan.

How to Maximize the Benefits of Exercises

Understanding the limitations of isometric exercises doesn't mean they're ineffective—it simply means they're most powerful when used appropriately. To get the most out of them:

1. Focus on Consistency

Regular practice is key. Aim for 3-4 sessions per week to see sustained benefits.

2. Pair with Stretching

Strengthening exercises should be balanced with stretches to maintain flexibility and prevent stiffness.

3. Monitor Progress

Keep track of how your body feels over time. Note improvements in posture, pain levels, or balance.

4. Seek Guidance

Consult a physical therapist to ensure you're performing exercises correctly and targeting the right muscle groups.

Realistic Expectations Lead to Better Results

It's easy to feel discouraged when exercises don't deliver immediate or dramatic results. However, scoliosis management is a long-term process. Isometric exercises may not "fix" your spine, but they can improve your quality of life, helping you move more freely, experience less pain, and feel stronger in your daily activities.

Strategic Suggestions

To navigate scoliosis effectively, surround yourself with a team of experts, including physical therapists, doctors, and supportive peers. Use isometric exercises as a foundation for managing your condition, and supplement them with other treatments as needed. This balanced approach ensures you're addressing scoliosis from every angle.

The Importance of Professional Guidance

Managing scoliosis can feel overwhelming, but you don't have to face it alone. Seeking professional guidance is one of the most important steps you can take to ensure your exercises and overall management plan are effective, safe, and tailored to your unique needs.

Why Professional Guidance Matters

Scoliosis is a complex condition that varies widely from person to person. No two spinal curves are identical, and the severity, location, and impact of the curve influence how your body functions. A professional, such as a physical therapist or a scoliosis specialist, has the expertise to assess your condition and create a personalized plan.

For example, while isometric exercises are beneficial, not all exercises are suitable for everyone. A professional can guide you in selecting movements that target your specific muscle imbalances and avoid placing undue stress on your spine. This ensures that your efforts are both effective and safe.

Customizing Your Exercise Routine

When it comes to scoliosis, a one-size-fits-all approach simply doesn't work. The exercises that benefit someone with a mild thoracic curve may not be appropriate for someone with a severe lumbar curve. Professionals take into account factors such as:

- The location and degree of your spinal curve
- Your age and stage of development
- Any associated symptoms, such as pain or limited mobility
- Your overall fitness level and health

For instance, a physical therapist might recommend side planks to strengthen your obliques if your scoliosis causes lateral imbalances. They may also suggest modifications, like using a pillow for support during wall sits, if you experience discomfort.

Preventing Injury and Overexertion

Without proper guidance, it's easy to unintentionally strain your back or perform exercises incorrectly. Even something as seemingly simple as a plank can lead to issues if your alignment is off or if you overdo it. Professionals provide valuable feedback to help you maintain proper form and avoid these pitfalls.

They can also help you progress gradually, increasing the intensity of your exercises as your strength improves. This reduces the risk of overexertion and ensures that your routine evolves with your abilities.

Integrating Exercises into a Broader Plan

Professional guidance goes beyond exercises. Experts can help you integrate isometric holds into a comprehensive scoliosis management plan that includes:

- **Stretching and Flexibility Work:** To address tight muscles that pull the spine out of alignment.
- **Aerobic Activity:** For overall health and endurance.
- **Postural Training:** To improve body awareness and balance.
- **Bracing or Medical Interventions:** If needed, based on the severity of your scoliosis.

Emotional Support and Motivation

Living with scoliosis can sometimes be emotionally challenging, particularly if pain or physical limitations interfere with your daily life. Professionals provide more than just technical expertise—they offer encouragement and reassurance that you're on the right path.

For instance, a physical therapist might celebrate small milestones with you, such as holding a plank for an extra 10 seconds or noticing an improvement in posture. This motivation can make a significant difference in sticking to your routine.

When and How to Seek Professional Help

You don't need to wait until scoliosis becomes severe to seek help. Consulting a professional early can prevent issues from worsening and set you up for success. Start by speaking with your doctor, who can refer you to a specialist, such as:

1. Physical Therapists

Experts in movement and rehabilitation, they can design and monitor an exercise program tailored to your needs.

2. Chiropractors

Some chiropractors specialize in scoliosis care, focusing on alignment and spinal health.

3. Orthopedic Specialists

They assess the structural aspects of scoliosis and may recommend bracing or other interventions if necessary.

Strategic Suggestions

Partnering with professionals gives you the confidence to navigate scoliosis effectively. Their guidance ensures your exercises are safe and impactful, helping you achieve lasting improvements. Build a strong support system that includes experts, and embrace the benefits of a tailored, well-rounded approach to scoliosis care.

Chapter 3: Core Isometric Exercises

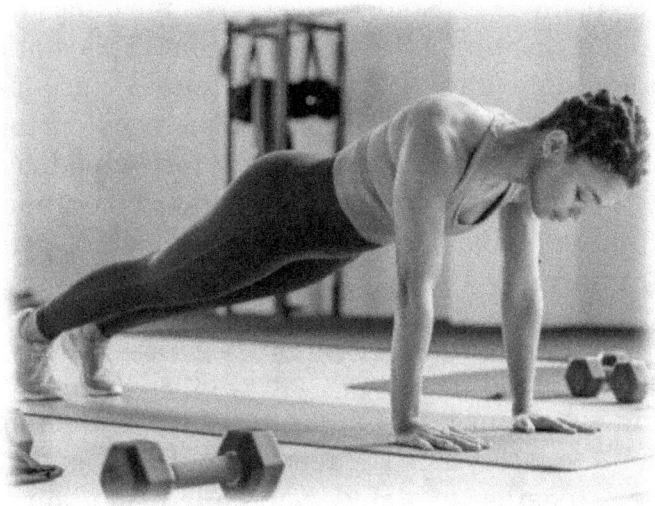

The plank is one of the most effective core exercises you can do, especially when it comes to managing scoliosis. It strengthens key muscle groups that help support your spine and improve your posture. When you incorporate different variations of the plank into your routine, you can target different muscles and progress at your own pace, ensuring maximum benefits for spinal stability and overall health.

Plank Variations for Core Stability

The plank is an isometric exercise, meaning you hold a position without movement. This static hold activates multiple muscle groups simultaneously, with a particular focus on the core. A strong core is essential for individuals with scoliosis because it helps support the spine, improves balance, and reduces the risk of pain or injury.

When you perform a plank, you engage muscles in your abdomen, lower back, hips, shoulders, and even your legs. For scoliosis, strengthening these muscles is particularly important, as they work together to stabilize and align your spine. Planks also promote better posture, which is key in managing scoliosis.

Common Plank Variations

Here are some plank variations that can be adjusted to your level of fitness and scoliosis severity, providing a progressive challenge while ensuring a safe approach to strengthening your core.

1. Standard Plank (Forearm Plank)

The forearm plank is the most basic form of the exercise and is great for beginners.

How to do it:

- Start in a push-up position, but with your forearms on the ground, elbows directly under your shoulders.
- Engage your core by drawing your belly button in towards your spine.
- Keep your body in a straight line from head to heels, avoiding sagging in your lower back or lifting your hips too high.
- Hold this position for 20-30 seconds or longer, depending on your strength level.

This variation provides an excellent foundation for building core strength. If you're new to planking, aim to hold this position for 15-30 seconds, gradually increasing the time as you gain strength.

2. High Plank (Push-Up Position)

The high plank is similar to the standard plank, but your arms are fully extended, supporting your body in a push-up position.

How to do it:

- Start in a push-up position, with your hands directly under your shoulders, fingers spread wide for better stability.
- Keep your body in a straight line, engaging your core and glutes to prevent your back from sagging.

- Hold the position for 20-30 seconds, focusing on maintaining good form.

The high plank challenges your shoulders and arms more than the forearm plank while still targeting your core. It can also help improve your wrist and shoulder mobility, which can be beneficial for individuals with scoliosis.

3. Plank with Leg Lifts

This variation adds an extra challenge to the traditional plank When you incorporate movement. Lifting one leg at a time engages the glutes and lower back, further strengthening the entire core.

How to do it:

- Start in a forearm plank position.
- Slowly lift one leg off the ground, keeping it straight and engaging your glutes.
- Hold for 3-5 seconds, then lower your leg and repeat on the other side.
- Alternate legs for 10-15 repetitions.

This variation helps activate the lower back and glutes, which are crucial for spinal stability in scoliosis. It also improves balance and coordination.

4. Side Plank

While side planks focus more on the oblique muscles, they're still an important plank variation for core stability and scoliosis management. Strengthening the sides of your core helps improve posture and balance, addressing muscle imbalances caused by scoliosis.

How to do it:

- Lie on your side with your forearm on the ground, elbow under your shoulder.
- Stack your feet or keep them staggered for more stability.
- Lift your hips off the ground, forming a straight line from your head to your feet.
- Hold for 20-30 seconds, then switch sides.

This exercise strengthens the obliques and can help reduce spinal curvature, especially when performed regularly.

5. Plank to Downward Dog

This variation combines the plank with a stretch, improving both core strength and flexibility.

How to do it:

- Start in a high plank position.
- Push your hips up toward the ceiling, forming an inverted "V" shape with your body.

- Hold for 2-3 seconds, then return to the high plank position.
- Repeat for 10-15 reps.

This variation challenges your core while offering a gentle stretch for your back, shoulders, and hamstrings. It can be especially beneficial if you experience tightness or stiffness due to scoliosis.

Progressing with Planks

As you become more comfortable with planking, you can gradually increase the duration of each hold, add more challenging variations, or incorporate other exercises into your routine to continue building strength. It's important to listen to your body and progress at a pace that feels comfortable.

Start with shorter intervals and work your way up. If you experience pain or discomfort, stop immediately and consult a professional to ensure your form is correct and you're not overexerting yourself.

Strategic Suggestions

To get the most out of plank variations, include them in a well-rounded exercise routine that addresses flexibility, strength, and cardiovascular health. Pair these planks with stretches, aerobic exercises, and other strength-training activities. Remember that consistency is key. Stick to your routine, and over time, you'll notice improvements in core stability, posture, and overall comfort.

Side Planks for Oblique Strength

Side planks are an excellent exercise for strengthening the oblique muscles, which are often underdeveloped in people with scoliosis. Strengthening these muscles is vital for improving spinal alignment, balance, and posture. Side planks offer a safe and effective way to work these key muscles without putting excessive strain on the back.

Why Focus on Obliques?

The oblique muscles are located on the sides of your torso, running diagonally from the ribcage to the pelvis. These muscles are responsible for stabilizing and rotating your torso, and they play a critical role in maintaining good posture and balance. In scoliosis, the spine may curve in ways that cause an imbalance in muscle strength and flexibility. Strengthening the obliques helps correct these imbalances by supporting the spine and improving its alignment.

A weak or imbalanced core can exacerbate the curvature of the spine, leading to pain, discomfort, and increased progression of the condition. Side planks target these critical oblique muscles, making them a powerful addition to your scoliosis management routine.

How to Perform the Side Plank

There are different variations of the side plank, which can be modified to suit your fitness level and scoliosis needs. Here's how to perform the standard side plank:

1. Start on Your Side

Lie on your side with your legs straight and your feet stacked on top of each other. Place your elbow directly beneath your shoulder, with your forearm resting on the floor for support.

2. Lift Your Hips

Engage your core by pulling your belly button toward your spine. Push your hips up, creating a straight line from your head to your feet. Be careful not to let your lower back sag or your hips drop toward the floor.

3. Hold the Position

Keep your body in a straight line and hold the position for 20-30 seconds. If you're a beginner, start with shorter intervals, gradually increasing the duration as you get stronger.

4. Lower and Repeat

Slowly lower your hips back to the ground and repeat on the other side. Aim for 2-3 sets per side.

Side planks are effective because they challenge your core stability while also targeting the sides of your torso. These muscles are often underutilized, especially in individuals with scoliosis, so strengthening them can lead to noticeable improvements in posture and spinal alignment.

Modifications for Beginners or Those with Scoliosis

If you're new to side planks or have scoliosis, you might find it challenging to hold the position for long periods. Here are some modifications to make the exercise more manageable while still targeting the oblique muscles:

1. Knee Down Side Plank

Instead of keeping both legs straight, bend the lower knee and place it on the floor for added stability. This modification reduces the intensity of the exercise while still engaging the oblique muscles.

2. Side Plank with Support

If you find it difficult to balance or keep your body straight, you can perform the side plank with your hand placed on a wall or sturdy piece of furniture. This extra support helps you focus on your form without worrying about balancing.

3. Side Plank with Leg Lift

As you gain strength, you can challenge yourself by lifting the top leg while holding the side plank position. This variation adds extra activation to the glutes and helps improve balance. To do this, lift your top leg slowly and hold it for a few seconds before lowering it back down.

4. Side Plank with Arm Extension

For a more advanced version, extend your top arm straight up toward the ceiling, creating a straight line from your hand to your feet. This variation challenges your balance and further activates the muscles in your core and shoulders.

Benefits of Side Planks for Scoliosis

Side planks help address muscle imbalances often caused by scoliosis. When your spine curves, it can create areas of weakness or tightness in certain muscles. Strengthening the obliques helps restore balance and provides better support for the spine. Here are the main benefits of side planks:

1. Improved Posture

Strengthening the obliques helps correct the postural distortions caused by scoliosis. With more balanced core muscles, your body is better aligned, leading to improved posture.

2. Reduced Pain

Stronger core muscles, including the obliques, can alleviate some of the pain caused by scoliosis, especially in the lower back and torso.

3. Enhanced Spinal Stability

Strengthening the obliques adds stability to the spine, which is particularly helpful for preventing further curvature and supporting the spine's alignment.

4. Better Balance

Strengthening the sides of the core improves balance, making it easier to move and perform daily tasks.

5. Prevention of Muscle Imbalances

Scoliosis can lead to uneven muscle strength, and side planks help address these imbalances by strengthening the weaker muscles.

How to Progress with Side Planks

As you build strength, you can gradually progress your side plank routine by increasing the duration of each hold, adding leg lifts or arm extensions, and performing more sets. However, it's essential to focus on form first.

If you're unable to hold the side plank for long periods, don't worry. Start with shorter intervals (e.g., 10-15 seconds) and gradually work your way up. Consistency is key when it comes to strengthening your obliques and improving spinal alignment.

Strategic Suggestions

Incorporating side planks into your daily routine can lead to significant improvements in spinal stability, posture, and pain management. Remember, it's essential to practice consistently and progress gradually. Combine side planks with other exercises to build a comprehensive scoliosis management plan. As you strengthen your core, you'll notice positive changes in your overall health and well-being.

Modified Planks for Beginners

Starting a core exercise routine can feel daunting, especially if you're dealing with scoliosis or have limited experience with physical activity. Modified planks are the perfect way to ease into core strengthening exercises while ensuring you maintain proper form and avoid strain. These beginner-friendly variations can help you build strength progressively, giving you the confidence to work toward more challenging plank positions in the future.

Why Modified Planks Are Important

For individuals with scoliosis, starting with modified planks can be an excellent way to ensure that your body is aligned correctly while still gaining the benefits of a strong, stable core. Traditional planks can be intense, and improper form may lead to discomfort or injury, especially if you are not used to engaging your core muscles. Modified planks allow you to perform the exercise in a way that feels safe and comfortable, focusing on building muscle endurance without overexertion.

Starting slow and working with modified planks also helps you avoid compensating with other muscle groups, such as your back, which can exacerbate your scoliosis. When you focus on proper form and building strength gradually, you can progress to more advanced variations when your body is ready.

Basic Modified Plank Variations

There are several modified plank variations that make it easier for beginners or those with scoliosis to engage the core muscles without overwhelming the body. Here's a breakdown of the most accessible options:

1. Knee Plank

The knee plank is one of the easiest ways to begin planking while still challenging your core. This variation reduces the intensity by keeping your knees on the ground instead of your toes, but it still targets the core and helps you build stability.

How to do it:

- Start in a traditional plank position, but lower your knees to the ground, keeping your feet off the floor.
- Ensure your hips are in line with your shoulders and knees to avoid sagging in the lower back.
- Engage your core by pulling your belly button toward your spine and hold the position for 15-30 seconds.
- Slowly lower and rest. Repeat for 2-3 sets.

This is a great starting point for building strength without placing too much pressure on your back or shoulders. As you progress, you can extend the time you hold the position and gradually shift to more challenging variations.

2. Wall Plank

If you find the floor plank too difficult, the wall plank is a great option for beginners. This modified plank variation allows you to engage your core while keeping your body at an angle, making it easier to hold the position for longer periods.

How to do it:

- Stand facing a wall and place your palms on the wall at shoulder height, about shoulder-width apart.
- Step back with your feet until you feel a slight angle in your body.
- Engage your core, keeping your body in a straight line from head to heels.
- Hold this position for 20-30 seconds, gradually increasing the duration as you build strength.
- Lower and rest between sets.

The wall plank is a gentler version that allows you to start strengthening your core with less intensity. It's particularly useful for people with scoliosis who may need extra support as they build muscle strength in their abdominal and back muscles.

3. Plank with Shoulder Taps

The plank with shoulder taps is a modified plank variation that targets the core while also improving shoulder stability. This exercise allows you to work your obliques, shoulders, and arms, which are all essential for stabilizing the spine in scoliosis management.

How to do it:

- Start in a knee plank position (as described above).
- Keep your body straight, and engage your core.
- Tap your right shoulder with your left hand while keeping your hips as still as possible.
- Return your left hand to the floor and repeat with the right hand to the left shoulder.
- Continue alternating for 10-12 reps on each side.

This exercise is excellent for beginners as it introduces dynamic movement to the plank while building stability and improving coordination. As you gain strength and stability, you can progress to more challenging plank variations.

4. Elevated Plank on an Exercise Ball

Using an exercise ball for an elevated plank is a great way to introduce an element of instability to your plank. This variation challenges your core without putting too much pressure on your back or shoulders. The ball adds a gentle balance challenge that helps improve coordination and engage deep core muscles.

How to do it:

- Start by placing your forearms on an exercise ball while keeping your knees on the ground.
- Ensure your body forms a straight line from your head to your knees.
- Engage your core, focusing on keeping your hips lifted and avoiding any sagging.
- Hold for 20-30 seconds, or as long as you feel comfortable.
- Rest and repeat for 2-3 sets.

Using an exercise ball increases the difficulty slightly offers great benefits for spinal stability and strengthening.

The Benefits of Modified Planks for Scoliosis

Modified planks provide an accessible way for individuals with scoliosis to start strengthening their core muscles while ensuring that their body stays aligned. Here are the key benefits:

1. Improved Spinal Stability

Modified planks strengthen the core muscles, providing support for the spine and reducing the risk of further curvature.

2. Reduced Risk of Injury

These variations reduce the intensity of traditional planks, making it easier to maintain proper form and avoid strain on the back or shoulders.

3. Building Core Strength Gradually

Starting with modified planks to gradually build up the necessary strength for more advanced exercises.

4. Enhanced Posture

Strengthening the core helps improve posture, reducing the misalignment caused by scoliosis and promoting better alignment throughout the day.

5. Pain Reduction

A strong core can help reduce discomfort and muscle imbalances associated with scoliosis.

How to Progress with Modified Planks

As you build core strength and endurance, you can begin to increase the difficulty of your modified planks. Start by increasing the hold time for each plank, adding variations like shoulder taps or leg lifts, and eventually transitioning to more advanced planks such as the standard forearm plank or high plank.

Remember to listen to your body and progress at your own pace. It's important to prioritize proper form over the duration or difficulty of the exercise. Consistency is key, and with regular practice, you'll notice improvements in your strength, posture, and overall comfort.

Strategic Suggestions

Modified planks are an excellent way to build the foundation of core strength needed for managing scoliosis. Stick to your routine, increase the intensity gradually, and combine planks with other exercises for a well-rounded approach to scoliosis care. Over time, you'll see improvements in your stability, posture, and pain management.

Chapter 4: Upper Body Isometric Exercises

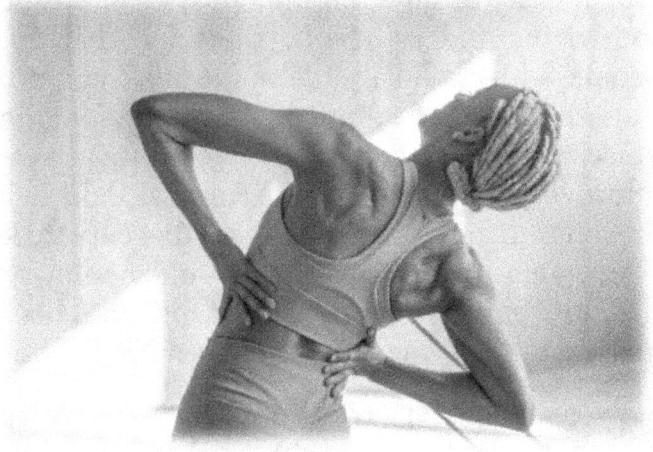

Wall push-ups are a fantastic way to build shoulder strength, especially if you're new to exercise or dealing with scoliosis. These modified push-ups are less intense than traditional ones but still offer a solid workout for the upper body. This exercise focuses on strengthening the shoulders, chest, and arms while engaging the core to maintain proper posture, making it an excellent addition to your scoliosis management routine.

Wall Push-Ups for Shoulder Strength

The muscles around the shoulders are crucial in supporting and stabilizing the upper back. In people with scoliosis, the spine may curve in ways that can lead to imbalances in the shoulder muscles. Strengthening these muscles can improve posture, reduce discomfort, and help prevent further progression of the curvature. Wall push-ups target the shoulder muscles without putting undue stress on the back, making them ideal for individuals with scoliosis.

Stronger shoulders contribute to better upper body alignment, which in turn helps support the spine. In people with scoliosis, weak shoulders can lead to uneven muscle activation, causing one shoulder to be higher than the other or contributing to the overall imbalance in posture. Wall push-ups help restore balance by strengthening both sides of the body equally.

How to Perform Wall Push-Ups

Here's how to do them properly:

1. Position Yourself Against a Wall

Stand facing a wall with your feet about shoulder-width apart. Place your hands flat against the wall, at about chest height and slightly wider than shoulder-width apart. The farther your feet are from the wall, the more challenging the exercise will be, so start with your feet closer for an easier version.

2. Engage Your Core

Before you begin, pull your belly button toward your spine to engage your core. Keeping your core activated will help you maintain proper posture and avoid straining your lower back.

3. Bend Your Elbows

Slowly bend your elbows and lower your chest toward the wall, keeping your body in a straight line from your head to your feet. Ensure that your elbows are going backward (not out to the sides) to keep your shoulder joints safe.

4. Push Back Up

Once your chest is close to the wall, push yourself back to the starting position by straightening your arms. Focus on using your chest and shoulder muscles to do the work, while maintaining stability in your core.

5. Repeat the Motion

Aim to perform 8-12 repetitions, depending on your fitness level. As you get stronger, you can increase the number of repetitions or move your feet farther from the wall to make the exercise more challenging.

Modifications for Wall Push-Ups

If you find wall push-ups too difficult at first, there are several ways to modify the exercise to suit your current strength level:

1. Feet Closer to the Wall

If you're finding it tough to complete a full range of motion, start by bringing your feet closer to the wall. This will make the push-up less intense and help you focus on building the necessary strength in your shoulders and chest.

2. Use a Softer Surface

If you're still getting used to the movement, try performing wall push-ups against a soft surface like a mattress or a cushioned mat. This can help reduce the intensity while still engaging your upper body.

3. Slow Down the Movement

If you're focusing on building strength, try slowing down the movement. Lower your body slowly toward the wall, hold the position for a few seconds, and then push back up at a slower pace. This increases the time under tension and helps build more muscle strength.

4. Incline Push-Ups

For an added challenge, you can perform wall push-ups with your hands on a higher surface (like the edge of a countertop or a sturdy table). This variation increases the angle, making the push-up harder while still providing support for your back.

Benefits of Wall Push-Ups for Scoliosis

Wall push-ups offer several key benefits that can improve overall posture and shoulder strength, especially for people with scoliosis:

1. Improved Shoulder Strength

Wall push-ups primarily target the shoulder muscles, helping to restore balance and strength to the upper body. Stronger shoulders support better posture and spinal alignment.

2. Enhanced Postural Alignment

Strengthening the shoulder muscles can improve your posture by promoting even muscle development on both sides of your upper body. This is especially important for scoliosis management.

3. Core Engagement

While the primary focus of wall push-ups is the upper body, your core muscles are also activated as you maintain a stable position. This dual activation improves both spinal stability and overall core strength.

4. Joint Protection

By performing wall push-ups instead of traditional floor push-ups, you reduce the strain on your wrists, elbows, and shoulders. This is particularly important for individuals with scoliosis who may already have an increased risk of joint stress.

5. Low-Impact Exercise

Wall push-ups are a low-impact exercise, making them accessible to individuals at different fitness levels and those with scoliosis. They don't put undue stress on the spine and are easier on the joints than floor push-ups.

How to Progress with Wall Push-Ups

As you get stronger, you can progressively increase the difficulty of your wall push-ups. Here are a few ways to challenge yourself:

1. Increase the Number of Repetitions

Start by performing 8-10 repetitions per set. As you build strength, aim to increase the number to 12-15 repetitions. The more you do, the stronger your shoulders will become.

2. Move Your Feet Backward

Gradually move your feet farther away from the wall. This will increase the angle of the push-up and make the exercise more challenging. Aim for a gradual increase in distance so that you don't strain your back or shoulders.

3. Add Variations

Once you are comfortable with basic wall push-ups, try adding variations to further challenge your shoulders. For example, you could try one-arm wall push-ups, or even include shoulder taps after each repetition to engage more stabilizing muscles.

4. Progress to Floor Push-Ups

When you feel ready, consider progressing to traditional push-ups on the floor. If you can perform several sets of wall push-ups with ease, floor push-ups will continue to build your shoulder strength and endurance.

Strategic Suggestions

Wall push-ups are a simple and effective exercise for improving shoulder strength and posture, especially when dealing with scoliosis. As you work through the variations and progressions, make sure to listen to your body and adjust the intensity as needed. Incorporate wall push-ups into your routine along with other exercises for a comprehensive approach to scoliosis management. With consistency, you'll notice significant improvements in your posture, strength, and overall comfort.

Isometric Rows for Back Muscles

Isometric rows are an excellent way to strengthen your back muscles, which play a vital role in supporting your spine, especially for individuals with scoliosis. These exercises target the upper back, shoulders, and arms, improving posture, stability, and muscle endurance. The beauty of isometric rows lies in their ability to engage the muscles without requiring dynamic movement, making them ideal for those who need to avoid excessive strain on their spine while still building strength.

Why Isometric Rows Are Important for Scoliosis

For individuals with scoliosis, the muscles along the back are often weakened or imbalanced due to the curvature of the spine. Strengthening these muscles can help stabilize the spine and reduce discomfort associated with uneven pressure on the back. Isometric rows specifically target the rhomboids, trapezius, and latissimus dorsi—muscles that help support the shoulders and upper back.

Isometric exercises, like rows, are particularly beneficial for people with scoliosis because they focus on muscle engagement without requiring excessive bending or twisting. The static hold of an isometric exercise strengthens muscles in a controlled manner, allowing for safe and effective training. Strengthening the back muscles through isometric rows can help correct posture imbalances, alleviate tension, and reduce the risk of injury as the body adapts to the curvature of the spine.

How to Perform Isometric Rows

Isometric rows require a resistance band or a cable machine, but you can also do them using simple household items like a towel or strap. Here's how to perform isometric rows with a resistance band:

1. Position Your Body

Stand tall with your feet shoulder-width apart, keeping a slight bend in your knees. Attach a resistance band to a sturdy object in front of you, such as a doorknob or a pole. Grasp the ends of the band with both hands, ensuring that the band is taut when your arms are extended in front of you.

2. Set Your Posture

Engage your core to support your spine and maintain a neutral posture throughout the movement. Imagine pulling your belly button toward your spine to activate the muscles in your abdomen. Keep your chest lifted and shoulders down, avoiding any hunching or rounding in your back.

3. Pull the Band Toward Your Chest

Start by pulling the band toward your chest, keeping your elbows close to your body. Focus on squeezing your shoulder blades together as you pull the band, engaging the muscles in your upper back and shoulders. This action mimics the motion of a rowing exercise but without the dynamic movement.

4. Hold the Position

Once your hands are close to your chest and your shoulder blades are squeezed together, hold this position for 10-30 seconds. Focus on maintaining good posture and keeping tension in the band throughout the hold.

5. Release and Repeat

Slowly release the tension in the band, returning your arms to the starting position. Rest briefly, then repeat for 2-3 sets, gradually increasing the hold time as your strength improves.

Modifications for Isometric Rows

If you're new to isometric exercises or have scoliosis, it's important to start with modifications that allow you to focus on form and avoid unnecessary strain. Here are some ways to adjust the exercise:

1. Use a Lighter Resistance Band

If you're just beginning, start with a resistance band that offers less tension. This will allow you to perform the exercise with good form while still engaging the muscles. As you get stronger, you can gradually increase the resistance by using a thicker band or adjusting the distance between your body and the anchor point.

2. Reduce the Hold Time

If holding the position for 30 seconds is too difficult, reduce the duration to 10 or 15 seconds. The key is to build strength progressively, so don't rush to extend the time before you're ready.

3. Adjust the Angle

If you're experiencing discomfort in your lower back or shoulders, adjust your body position. You can perform the exercise seated or standing at a less intense angle to reduce strain. The goal is to maintain a stable posture without overexerting yourself.

4. Use a Towel or Strap

If you don't have a resistance band, you can perform a similar isometric row using a towel or strap. Secure one end of the towel to a stationary object and hold both ends of the towel with your hands. Pull the towel toward you, holding the contraction for several seconds.

Benefits of Isometric Rows for Scoliosis

Isometric rows offer several benefits, especially for individuals with scoliosis. Strengthening the upper back and shoulder muscles helps improve posture, enhance spinal stability, and reduce pain and discomfort. Here's how isometric rows can be beneficial for scoliosis:

1. Improved Posture

Strengthening the muscles that support your back can help correct postural imbalances associated with scoliosis. Stronger muscles in the upper back encourage better spinal alignment, helping to reduce the effects of the curvature.

2. Increased Spinal Stability

The back muscles play a key role in stabilizing the spine. When you strengthen these muscles, you increase overall spinal stability, which can help prevent further curvature and alleviate discomfort.

3. Reduced Risk of Injury

Isometric rows strengthen the muscles around the spine and shoulders, making them more resilient to injury. When these muscles are weak or imbalanced, it can lead to increased strain on the spine and surrounding structures.

4. No Dynamic Movement Required

Since isometric rows involve holding a static position rather than dynamic movement, they are less likely to aggravate the spine or cause pain in individuals with scoliosis. The exercise allows you to build strength safely.

5. Low-Impact Exercise

Isometric exercises are low-impact, which means they won't put undue stress on the joints or spine. This makes them ideal for people with scoliosis who need to avoid high-impact exercises.

How to Progress with Isometric Rows

Here are some ways to progress:

1. Increase the Hold Time

Start by holding for 10-15 seconds, and gradually increase to 30-60 seconds as your endurance improves. Longer hold times provide more time for muscle activation, helping you build strength.

2. Increase Resistance

Gradually increase the tension in the band or use a thicker band. This adds resistance, making the exercise more challenging and helping you build stronger muscles.

3. **Perform More Sets**

If you're currently doing 2-3 sets, try adding more sets to your routine. Adding an extra set or two will help build muscle endurance and strength over time.

3. **Combine with Other Upper Body Exercises:**

For a more comprehensive upper body workout, combine isometric rows with other upper body exercises like wall push-ups or resistance band chest presses. This will target different muscle groups for a well-rounded approach to strengthening the upper body.

Strategic Suggestions

Isometric rows are an excellent way to strengthen the muscles that support your spine and shoulders, particularly for people with scoliosis. When you incorporate them into your routine and progressing at your own pace, you'll build strength, improve posture, and reduce discomfort. Stay consistent, and remember that gradual progress is key to achieving long-term benefits.

Resistance Band Holds for Upper Body Balance

Resistance band holds are another highly effective way to strengthen your upper body and improve your balance, especially when managing scoliosis. These isometric exercises engage multiple muscle groups, including the shoulders, arms, and upper back, while encouraging stability in the body. With resistance band holds, you can effectively target key muscles that support your posture and spinal alignment, which is particularly important for individuals with scoliosis.

Why Focus on Upper Body Balance for Scoliosis?

One of the challenges of scoliosis is the imbalance it creates between the muscles on each side of the body. This can lead to uneven muscle strength and poor posture. Strengthening the muscles in the upper body—particularly the shoulders, upper back, and arms—can help balance these disparities, reduce pain, and promote a more aligned spine. Resistance band holds help activate these muscles in a controlled, low-impact way.

Upper body balance is crucial for scoliosis management because it provides better support for the spine. A balanced upper body can help reduce the compensations the body makes due to an uneven curvature, helping to align the spine more effectively. These exercises can also help reduce the risk of other postural issues that can arise from the muscular imbalances caused by scoliosis.

How to Perform Resistance Band Holds

Performing resistance band holds is straightforward, and you can do them at home with minimal equipment. Here's how to get started:

1. Choose Your Resistance Band

Select a resistance band with the appropriate tension for your fitness level. A light or medium resistance band is ideal for beginners, but as you get stronger, you can increase the tension. Make sure the band is securely anchored to a sturdy object, like a door or a heavy piece of furniture, or you can hold both ends of the band in your hands.

2. Set Your Starting Position

Stand with your feet shoulder-width apart. Hold the resistance band with both hands, either in front of your body or to the side, depending on the variation you are doing. If you are working on shoulder strength, pull the band horizontally; if you're targeting your back or chest, you can adjust the band to perform other variations.

3. Activate Your Core and Shoulders

Before you start the exercise, activate your core by gently pulling your belly button toward your spine. Keep your chest open and your shoulders down and back. Engage your upper back muscles to prepare for the hold.

4. Hold the Band in Place

Pull the band apart slightly to create tension, then hold it in place. Keep your arms extended straight in front of you or out to the sides, depending on the type of resistance band hold you're doing. Make sure your body stays aligned and stable—avoid arching your back or shrugging your shoulders.

5. Maintain the Position

Hold the position for 15-30 seconds, depending on your strength level. Focus on maintaining tension in the band while keeping your core and upper body stable. Avoid letting your posture slip, and breathe deeply as you hold the position.

6. Release and Repeat

After holding the position for the designated time, slowly release the tension in the band and rest. Repeat the exercise for 2-3 sets, gradually increasing the hold time as you build strength.

Modifications for Resistance Band Holds

Here are a few ways to modify the resistance band holds if you find them too challenging:

1. Use a Lighter Resistance Band

If you're new to resistance training or dealing with scoliosis, choose a resistance band that offers light tension. This allows you to focus on form and control without straining your muscles.

2. Shorten the Hold Time

Start with shorter holds, around 10-15 seconds, and gradually increase the duration as your muscles get stronger. As you build endurance, you can hold for longer periods, up to 30 seconds or more.

3. Perform the Hold with a Different Angle

If you find it difficult to hold the band at shoulder height or out to the sides, try performing the exercise at a lower angle to reduce the intensity. As you get stronger, you can increase the difficulty by adjusting the angle at which you hold the band.

4. Seated Variation

If standing is difficult for you, try performing the resistance band hold while seated. This allows you to focus on your upper body without worrying about balance. Sit in a sturdy chair with your feet flat on the ground, and hold the resistance band as you would in the standing position.

Benefits of Resistance Band Holds for Scoliosis

Resistance band holds offer a variety of benefits, especially for those managing scoliosis. This exercise targets key muscle groups and helps improve muscle engagement, endurance, and overall spinal alignment. Here are some specific benefits:

1. Improved Postural Control

Resistance band holds engage muscles that stabilize the upper body, which helps improve posture. Strengthening these muscles promotes more even alignment of the spine and reduces the risk of postural imbalances.

2. Strengthened Shoulder and Upper Back Muscles

Holding a resistance band in a stable position strengthens the muscles of the upper back, shoulders, and arms. These muscles help support the spine and reduce the strain caused by scoliosis.

3. Core Engagement

While focusing on the upper body, resistance band holds also activate the core muscles. Maintaining proper posture during the hold strengthens the abdominal muscles, which play an important role in supporting the spine.

4. Low-Impact Exercise

Resistance band holds are a low-impact exercise, making them suitable for individuals with scoliosis who need to avoid high-impact activities. These exercises strengthen muscles safely and effectively without putting stress on the spine.

5. Enhanced Balance and Stability

Holding the resistance band in place requires stability and control, which improves overall balance. This is especially beneficial for people with scoliosis, as it helps correct uneven muscle activation and promotes more balanced movements.

How to Progress with Resistance Band Holds

As you get stronger, it's important to challenge yourself by gradually increasing the difficulty of the exercise. Here are some ways to progress:

1. Increase the Hold Time

As you build strength and endurance, try to hold the band for longer periods. Start with 15 seconds and gradually increase the duration to 30-60 seconds. The longer you hold, the more endurance you build in your muscles.

2. Increase Resistance

As you get stronger, you can move to a heavier resistance band. A stronger band will increase the tension and make the exercise more challenging. Be sure to maintain proper form as the intensity increases.

3. Add More Sets

Start with 2-3 sets, and as you progress, aim to add more sets to your routine. Performing 4-5 sets of resistance band holds will help improve overall strength and endurance.

4. Try Different Variations

Once you're comfortable with basic resistance band holds, you can try other variations to target different muscle groups. You can do front and side raises, or combine holds with other movements to challenge your upper body.

Strategic Suggestions

Resistance band holds are a great exercise for building upper body strength, balance, and stability, especially for people with scoliosis. When you perform these exercises regularly, you'll improve muscle endurance, support better posture, and strengthen the muscles that help stabilize your spine. Stay consistent with your practice and gradually increase the intensity as your body adapts. The key is to progress at your own pace, ensuring that you build strength without overstraining your body.

Chapter 5: Lower Body Isometric Exercises

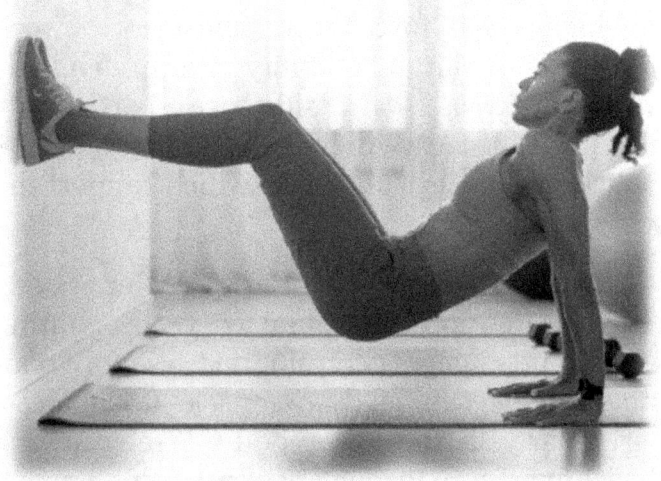

Wall sits are an excellent exercise to strengthen your lower body muscles, especially for those managing scoliosis. This simple yet effective isometric exercise targets the quads, hamstrings, and glutes, helping to build muscle endurance and stability. Wall sits not only contribute to overall leg strength but also improve postural support, making them a vital part of your scoliosis exercise routine.

Wall Sits for Leg Strength

A wall sit is a static exercise where you hold a seated position against a wall for an extended period. The key is to hold this position without moving, which forces your muscles to work harder to maintain stability. For individuals with scoliosis, wall sits are particularly beneficial because they help strengthen the muscles in the legs and core, which support the spine.

When you have scoliosis, your body compensates for the spinal curve by shifting weight and engaging certain muscles more than others. This can lead to muscle imbalances, particularly in the lower body. Strengthening the legs and core through wall sits helps create a more balanced foundation for the spine. When you improve the stability of your lower body, you reduce the strain placed on your back, which can alleviate pain and improve posture over time.

How to Perform a Wall Sit

Performing a wall sit correctly is essential to getting the most out of the exercise and avoiding injury. Here's a step-by-step guide to help you set up and execute a wall sit:

1. Find a Flat Wall

Start by standing with your back flat against a wall. Your feet should be about 12-18 inches away from the wall, and your feet should be shoulder-width apart.

2. Slide Down into Position

Slowly slide your back down the wall, bending your knees until your thighs are parallel to the ground. Your knees should be directly over your ankles, forming a 90-degree angle. Your hips should also be level with your knees, and your back should remain flat against the wall. Avoid arching your lower back.

3. Engage Your Core

While holding this position, focus on engaging your core. Gently pull your belly button towards your spine to activate your abdominal muscles. This will provide additional stability and support for your lower back.

4. Hold the Position

Once you are in the correct position, hold the wall sit for a set amount of time. Beginners can start with 15-20 seconds, gradually increasing the duration as they build strength. Keep your knees aligned with your toes and avoid letting them extend past your feet.

5. Breath and Relax

During the wall sit, remember to breathe deeply and steadily. Avoid holding your breath, as this can create unnecessary tension. If you feel any discomfort or strain in your knees or back, stop the exercise and reassess your form.

6. Slowly Stand Up

When you're ready to finish, slowly slide back up the wall to a standing position. Take a moment to rest before attempting another set.

Modifications for Wall Sits

If you're new to wall sits or experiencing difficulty maintaining the position, there are several ways to modify the exercise:

1. Shorten the Hold Time

If holding the wall sit for an extended period feels challenging, start with shorter intervals. Try holding the position for 10-15 seconds and gradually build up your endurance.

2. Support Your Back

For extra support, you can place a small cushion or towel behind your lower back. This can help you maintain the proper form without straining the muscles in your back.

3. Shallow Wall Sits

If a full wall sit feels too intense, try a modified, shallow wall sit where your knees don't bend as deeply. This will reduce the amount of stress placed on your legs and make it easier to hold the position.

4. Use a Stability Ball

For a more advanced version, you can perform wall sits with a stability ball placed between your lower back and the wall. The ball adds an extra challenge by requiring additional engagement from your core and stabilizing muscles.

5. Assisted Wall Sit

For beginners, it may help to perform the wall sit with the assistance of a chair or other support. This allows you to focus on form and gradually work up to holding the position independently.

Benefits of Wall Sits for Scoliosis

Wall sits are more than just a lower body exercise; they provide a range of benefits that are particularly useful for those with scoliosis:

1. Stronger Lower Body Muscles

Wall sits primarily target the quadriceps, hamstrings, and glutes, which are all essential muscles for supporting the lower back and pelvis. Strengthening these muscles can improve posture and reduce discomfort in the spine caused by muscle imbalances.

2. Core Stability

Maintaining a wall sit requires significant core activation. Engaging your core throughout the exercise strengthens the muscles around your spine, promoting better alignment and stability.

3. Improved Posture

Strengthening the lower body and core helps to stabilize the entire body. This improved stability reduces the tendency to slouch or shift weight unevenly, which is common with scoliosis. Over time, this can improve your overall posture.

4. Increased Endurance

Wall sits are an isometric exercise, meaning you hold the position without movement. This type of exercise builds muscle endurance, allowing your muscles to work for longer periods without tiring. Increased endurance helps your body perform everyday activities with less effort and discomfort.

5. Low-Impact Exercise

Wall sits are a low-impact exercise, making them suitable for people with scoliosis who need to avoid high-impact or stressful movements. They are gentle on the joints while still offering significant strength-building benefits.

How to Progress with Wall Sits

Once you're comfortable with the basic wall sit, you can progress in several ways to continue building strength and endurance:

1. Increase Hold Time

As you build strength, aim to increase the duration of your wall sit. Start with 30 seconds and work your way up to 1-2 minutes per set.

2. Add Weight

For a more challenging variation, you can add weight to your wall sit. Hold a dumbbell or kettlebell in your lap to increase the intensity and further challenge your leg muscles.

3. Advanced Wall Sit Variations

Once you're comfortable with the basic wall sit, try incorporating leg lifts or alternating knee raises while holding the position. These variations increase the difficulty by engaging the core and hip muscles.

4. Perform Multiple Sets

As you become more advanced, aim to perform multiple sets of wall sits. Start with 2-3 sets and gradually increase to 4-5 sets, taking short breaks in between.

Strategic Suggestions

Wall sits are a highly effective exercise for building leg strength, improving posture, and stabilizing the lower body, particularly for individuals with scoliosis. Consistency is key in seeing results. Make wall sits a regular part of your routine, and gradually increase the difficulty as you get stronger. Doing so will enhance your muscle endurance, promote better posture, and reduce discomfort in your spine over time.

Glute Bridges for Hip Stability

Glute bridges are an excellent isometric exercise that focuses on the glutes, hips, and lower back, making them a vital part of a scoliosis exercise routine. These exercises strengthen the muscles responsible for stabilizing your pelvis and spine, helping correct muscle imbalances, reduce pain, and improve overall posture. Glute bridges are simple but powerful, targeting the muscles needed for effective spinal support.

What Is a Glute Bridge and How Does It Help with Scoliosis?

A glute bridge is an exercise where you lift your hips off the ground while keeping your feet planted. The movement primarily engages the gluteus muscles, but it also works the lower back, hamstrings, and core. This exercise is particularly important for scoliosis because many individuals with scoliosis have weak glute and hip muscles. Weakness in these muscles can cause uneven pressure on the spine, exacerbating the spinal curve or contributing to poor posture.

When you strengthen the glutes and hips, you create a solid base of support for the spine. The glute bridge helps to activate these muscles, leading to better spinal alignment and reducing the risk of further curvature or discomfort. Additionally, this exercise improves your overall posture, enhances movement patterns, and stabilizes the pelvis.

How to Perform a Glute Bridge

Performing a glute bridge is straightforward, but it requires careful attention to form to ensure you're activating the right muscles and avoiding unnecessary strain:

1. Set Up Your Position

Start by lying flat on your back with your knees bent and feet hip-width apart. Place your feet about 12 inches from your hips, keeping your heels flat on the ground. Your arms should be extended at your sides with your palms facing down.

2. Engage Your Core and Glutes

Before you lift your hips, engage your core muscles. Tighten your abdominal muscles by gently pulling your belly button toward your spine. At the same time, squeeze your glutes to prepare them for the lift.

3. Lift Your Hips

Press through your heels and lift your hips off the ground towards the ceiling. Your body should form a straight line from your shoulders to your knees at the top of the movement. Avoid overextending your back—focus on using your glutes and hamstrings to lift your hips.

4. Pause at the Top

Hold the bridge position at the top for a second or two. During this pause, make sure your glutes are fully engaged and your core remains tight. Avoid letting your lower back arch too much, as this can lead to unnecessary strain.

5. Lower Slowly

Slowly lower your hips back down toward the floor, keeping control of the movement. Don't let your lower back or hips sag as you descend—maintain engagement of your glutes and core.

6. Repeat the Movement

Aim to perform 10-15 repetitions for beginners, focusing on slow and controlled movements. Over time, you can increase the number of reps or sets as you build strength.

Modifications for Glute Bridges

If you're new to glute bridges or experiencing difficulty with the movement, there are several ways to modify the exercise to fit your needs:

1. Increase Hold Time

Instead of focusing on repetitions, you can increase the hold time at the top of the movement. Start with holding for 3-5 seconds and gradually increase the duration as you build strength.

2. Glute Bridge with Marching

For a more challenging variation, you can add a marching movement at the top of the bridge. Once your hips are lifted, alternate lifting one knee towards your chest, keeping the hips stable. This variation increases the demand on your core and hip flexors.

3. Single-Leg Glute Bridges

A more advanced modification is performing the glute bridge with one leg raised. Lift one leg off the ground while keeping the other planted, and then perform the same movement.

4. Use a Stability Ball

Another variation involves placing your feet on a stability ball instead of the floor. This forces your core and glute muscles to work harder to stabilize your body during the lift.

5. Elevated Glute Bridge

If you're comfortable with the standard glute bridge, you can try elevating your feet on a bench or platform. This increases the range of motion, which intensifies the exercise.

Benefits of Glute Bridges for Scoliosis

Glute bridges are not only effective at targeting the glutes and hamstrings, but they also offer a number of benefits that are crucial for managing scoliosis:

1. Improved Hip Stability

Glute bridges strengthen the muscles that support the pelvis, including the glutes and hip flexors. For those with scoliosis, hip instability can contribute to spinal misalignment. Strengthening these muscles helps prevent compensatory movements and improves overall stability.

2. Spinal Alignment

By engaging the glutes and core, glute bridges help stabilize the pelvis and support the spine. This stabilization improves spinal alignment, which can reduce the degree of curvature over time and alleviate discomfort associated with scoliosis.

3. Increased Core Strength

The glute bridge is also an effective way to engage your core muscles, which play a vital role in supporting your spine. Strengthening your core provides better spinal support and reduces the likelihood of back pain.

4. Postural Improvement

Regularly performing glute bridges can contribute to better posture. When the glutes and core muscles are strong, it becomes easier to maintain a neutral pelvis and spine, reducing the likelihood of slouching or misalignment.

5. Muscle Balance

People with scoliosis often experience muscle imbalances due to the uneven distribution of weight and pressure on the body. Glute bridges help balance these muscle groups by strengthening the posterior chain, which includes the glutes, hamstrings, and lower back. A balanced muscle structure promotes better movement patterns and reduces strain on the spine.

How to Progress with Glute Bridges

Once you are comfortable with the basic glute bridge, you can increase the intensity and challenge your muscles further by progressing the exercise:

1. Increase Reps and Sets

Start by performing 2-3 sets of 10-15 reps, gradually increasing the number of sets and reps as you gain strength. Aim for 4-5 sets as you advance.

2. Add Resistance

To make the glute bridge more challenging, you can add resistance by holding a weight plate or dumbbell over your hips. This will increase the intensity and further activate the glute and hamstring muscles.

3. Perform Slow and Controlled Movements

To maximize muscle engagement, perform the glute bridge with slow, controlled movements. Focus on squeezing your glutes at the top and slowly lowering your hips to the ground. This slower tempo will help build strength more effectively.

4. Incorporate Variations

As you progress, add variations to keep the exercise challenging. Try single-leg bridges, elevated bridges, or glute bridges with marching for a more dynamic workout.

Strategic Suggestions

Glute bridges are an essential exercise for strengthening the muscles around the hips and spine. When you make them a regular part of your routine, you can help stabilize the pelvis, reduce pain, and improve overall spinal alignment. Stay consistent and gradually increase the difficulty as your muscles become stronger. This will not only benefit your scoliosis management but also enhance your overall posture and strength.

Isometric Lunges for Muscle Imbalance Correction

Isometric lunges are an excellent exercise for correcting muscle imbalances and improving lower body strength, particularly for those managing scoliosis. This exercise works by engaging the major muscle groups in the legs and hips, helping to restore balance in the body and stabilize the pelvis and spine. Isometric lunges, which involve holding the lunge position without movement, provide a low-impact way to build strength, improve posture, and correct asymmetries in the body caused by scoliosis.

What Are Isometric Lunges and How Do They Help with Scoliosis?

An isometric lunge is a variation of the traditional lunge where you hold the lunge position instead of moving up and down. The focus is on maintaining a static position with the muscles engaged, which allows for more time under tension and deeper muscle activation. This exercise targets the quads, hamstrings, glutes, and hip stabilizers, all of which are essential for proper posture and spinal alignment.

For people with scoliosis, muscle imbalances are common due to the uneven forces on the body caused by the spinal curve. Many people with scoliosis have one leg that may be slightly stronger or more active than the other, leading to muscle imbalances that affect posture and increase strain on the spine. Isometric lunges can help address these imbalances by strengthening both legs equally, providing more stability to the pelvis and spine, and promoting better posture.

Holding the lunge position also forces you to focus on core activation and stabilization. A strong, engaged core is essential for scoliosis management because it helps support the spine and reduces the risk of injury or discomfort.

How to Perform Isometric Lunges

Here's a step-by-step guide to help you perform this exercise correctly:

1. Start in a Standing Position

Begin by standing tall with your feet hip-width apart. Make sure your shoulders are relaxed, and your core is engaged. You can keep your hands on your hips, or for added balance, you can place them in front of you.

2. Step Into a Lunge

Take a step forward with your right foot and bend both knees to drop into a lunge. The front knee should be bent at a 90-degree angle, with your knee directly above your ankle. The back knee should hover just above the floor, and your back leg should be bent at about 90 degrees as well.

3. Hold the Position

Once you're in the lunge position, hold it for a set period of time. Try to hold for 20-30 seconds to start, and gradually increase the time as you build strength and endurance. Ensure your torso remains upright, with your shoulders stacked over your hips and your back straight. Engage your core and squeeze your glutes to support your pelvis.

4. Check Your Alignment

Keep your knee from extending past your toes in the front leg. Ensure your back leg is also in a 90-degree angle, not too straight or too bent. Make sure your hips are square and your knees are aligned with your toes.

5. Switch Sides

After holding the lunge on one leg for the desired amount of time, return to a standing position and repeat the same movement on the opposite leg. Perform 2-3 sets on each side, holding the position for 20-30 seconds per side.

Modifications for Isometric Lunges

If you are new to lunges or find them challenging due to balance or strength limitations, there are several modifications you can try to make the exercise more manageable:

1. Use a Wall or Chair for Support

To help with balance, you can place your hand on a wall or chair as you hold the lunge position. This will provide extra stability and allow you to focus on proper form and muscle engagement.

2. Shorten the Lunge Step

If stepping too far forward feels uncomfortable, try shortening your lunge. A smaller step will still target the quads and glutes but may feel more stable and manageable.

3. Lower the Duration

Start with holding the lunge position for 10-15 seconds, and gradually increase the time as your endurance improves. Holding for a few seconds will still provide muscle activation and benefit.

4. Elevate the Back Leg

To increase the difficulty of the lunge, try elevating your back leg on a small step or platform. This modification requires more stability from the hip and core, making the exercise more challenging.

5. Use a Cushion or Mat

If your knees feel uncomfortable on the ground during the exercise, place a cushion or exercise mat under your knees to provide extra padding and support.

Benefits of Isometric Lunges for Scoliosis

Isometric lunges offer numerous benefits for individuals with scoliosis. Here are some key advantages:

1. Improved Muscle Imbalance Correction

One of the primary benefits of isometric lunges is their ability to correct muscle imbalances. When you hold the lunge position, you strengthen both legs evenly, addressing any discrepancies between the left and right sides of the body. This helps correct uneven muscle strength that often occurs with scoliosis, promoting better posture and alignment.

2. Enhanced Core Stability

Holding a lunge position requires significant core engagement. A strong core is crucial for people with scoliosis, as it helps support the spine and maintain good posture.

3. Increased Lower Body Strength

Isometric lunges target the major muscles of the lower body, including the glutes, quads, hamstrings, and calves. Strengthening these muscles is vital for stabilizing the pelvis and supporting the spine. The more balanced and strong your lower body muscles are, the less strain you place on your back.

4. Improved Posture

Isometric lunges can improve overall posture. The exercise encourages the activation of the glutes and core, which helps stabilize the spine and reduce the risk of slumping or misalignment.

5. Low-Impact Exercise

Isometric lunges are a low-impact exercise, making them suitable for individuals with scoliosis who may be wary of high-impact movements. When you hold the lunge position, you still achieve significant muscle activation without causing excessive strain on the joints.

6. Better Hip Stability

Isometric lunges engage the hip stabilizers, helping to improve hip stability and prevent excessive tilting or rotation of the pelvis.

How to Progress with Isometric Lunges

As you become more comfortable with isometric lunges, you can increase the intensity and duration to continue building strength and stability:

1. Increase the Hold Time

Start by holding each lunge position for 20-30 seconds and gradually increase the time to 45 seconds or longer as your strength improves.

2. Add Weighted Resistance

For added intensity, hold a dumbbell or kettlebell in each hand while performing the lunge. This will make the exercise more challenging.

3. Increase the Number of Sets

As you progress, try adding more sets to your routine. Start with 2-3 sets per leg, and work up to 4-5 sets as you become stronger.

4. Try Pulse Lunges

Add pulses to the lunge by gently lowering your hips up and down a few inches while holding the position. This will add an extra challenge and increase muscle activation.

5. Perform on an Elevated Surface

Perform isometric lunges with one foot elevated on a step or platform. This will require greater stability from your lower body and core.

Strategic Suggestions

Isometric lunges are a powerful exercise for correcting muscle imbalances and improving lower body stability. As with all exercises, consistency is key to seeing results. Keep practicing the movement, and remember that progress takes time. Focus on your form, gradually increase your hold time, and challenge yourself with progressions to continue building strength and improving posture. As you strengthen your legs and core, you will notice better spinal alignment and reduced discomfort related to scoliosis. Stay committed, and be patient with your progress.

Chapter 6: Postural and Spine-Supportive Isometric Exercises

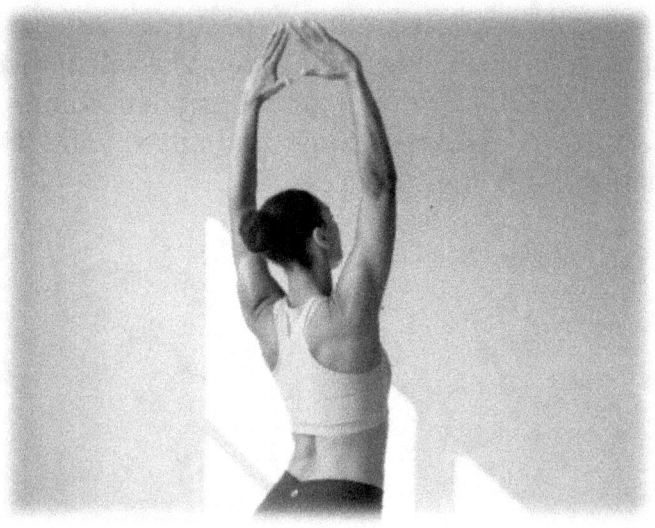

Wall Angels are a simple but effective isometric exercise designed to improve your posture, strengthen your shoulders, and promote spinal health. They are especially beneficial for individuals with scoliosis, as they help increase mobility in the upper back and shoulders, areas that can become stiff or misaligned due to the curve of the spine. This exercise is particularly useful in combating rounded shoulders and forward head posture, which are common issues for people dealing with scoliosis. When you practice Wall Angels, you can encourage a more natural alignment of your spine and improve overall posture.

Wall Angels for Improved Posture

Wall Angels are a posture-correcting exercise that involves standing with your back against a wall while moving your arms in a controlled motion, mimicking the movement of snow angels. This simple motion helps open up the chest, stretch the shoulder muscles, and strengthen the upper back. The key is that the movement is done while maintaining contact with the wall, which ensures that your spine stays aligned and that your body doesn't compensate by leaning or arching.

For people with scoliosis, especially those with a thoracic (mid-back) curve, the muscles surrounding the upper back, shoulders, and neck may be weak or tense. Wall Angels help to relieve this tension, stretch tight muscles, and strengthen the ones that are underactive. When performed regularly, Wall Angels can be a great tool for improving posture, which can also reduce back pain and improve overall spinal health.

How to Perform Wall Angels

To get the most out of Wall Angels, it's important to perform them correctly. Here's a step-by-step guide:

1. Start with Your Back Against the Wall

Stand with your back flat against the wall. Make sure your feet are about 4 to 6 inches away from the base of the wall, so that your lower back is touching the wall but not overly arched. You should feel a natural curve in your lower back, but your back should remain in contact with the wall.

2. Position Your Arms

Bring your arms up so your elbows are bent at a 90-degree angle. Your upper arms should be parallel to the ground, and your forearms should be perpendicular to your upper arms, like the shape of a "W". Press your arms, wrists, and elbows into the wall as much as possible. If you can't keep your arms fully in contact with the wall, don't worry—just try your best to get as close as possible. This will improve over time with practice.

3. Engage Your Core

Before starting the movement, engage your core muscles to protect your lower back. Drawing your belly button toward your spine will help keep your spine in a neutral position and prevent arching.

4. Move Your Arms Slowly

Keeping your arms in the "W" position, slowly slide them upward along the wall, aiming to form a "Y" shape with your arms. Try to maintain contact with the wall throughout the motion. Lift your arms as high as you can without losing contact with the wall or arching your back. It's important to keep your shoulders down, away from your ears, throughout the movement.

5. Hold and Return to the Starting Position

Once you have reached the highest position that you can, hold for a few seconds (around 5-10 seconds). Then, slowly slide your arms back down to the starting position in the "W" shape.

6. Repeat the Movement

Perform 8-12 repetitions, holding each position at the top for a few seconds. Start with 1-2 sets and increase as you become more comfortable with the movement.

Modifications and Tips for Wall Angels

If you find Wall Angels difficult at first, don't worry—there are several modifications you can try to make the exercise more accessible:

1. Start with Less Range of Motion

If you can't keep your arms fully against the wall, start by performing the movement within a smaller range. Don't force your arms higher than what feels comfortable. As you continue practicing, your range of motion will naturally improve.

2. Use a Pillow or Cushion for Your Lower Back

If you find that your lower back is arching too much during the exercise, try placing a small cushion or pillow between your lower back and the wall. This will help you keep your spine in a neutral position while still engaging the muscles of your back and shoulders.

3. Try with a Stability Ball

To make the exercise more challenging, you can perform Wall Angels with a stability ball positioned against your upper back. This adds an element of instability and helps to strengthen the stabilizing muscles around your shoulder blades and spine.

4. Progress by Increasing Hold Time

Once you are comfortable with the Wall Angels, try holding the top position for longer periods of time, such as 15-20 seconds. This will further challenge your shoulder muscles and improve strength.

5. Perform with a Partner or Trainer

If you're unsure about your form, consider having a partner or trainer assist you. They can help ensure that your arms and spine are aligned correctly during the movement.

Benefits of Wall Angels for Scoliosis

Wall Angels offer several key benefits, particularly for people with scoliosis. Here are some reasons why this exercise is so effective:

1. Improved Posture

Wall Angels help open up the chest and activate the muscles in your upper back, encouraging better posture. For those with scoliosis, improving posture can reduce the strain on the spine and minimize discomfort.

2. Shoulder and Upper Back Strength

The movement of Wall Angels strengthens the muscles of the shoulders, upper back, and neck. Stronger shoulders and upper back muscles can help support the spine, reducing the risk of slumping or rounding your shoulders.

3. Increased Flexibility

By regularly performing Wall Angels, you can improve your range of motion in the shoulders and upper back. This is particularly helpful for individuals with scoliosis who may have stiffness in these areas due to muscle imbalances or the curvature of the spine.

4. Reduced Neck and Upper Back Tension

Many people with scoliosis experience tension and discomfort in the neck and upper back, particularly due to poor posture. Wall Angels help alleviate some of this tension by promoting proper alignment and stretching tight muscles.

5. Core Engagement

While focusing on the arms and upper body, Wall Angels also engage your core muscles to maintain stability and proper posture. A strong core is essential for people with scoliosis, as it provides support to the spine and helps prevent further misalignment.

6. Low-Impact and Accessible

Wall Angels are a low-impact exercise, making them suitable for people at various fitness levels, including those with scoliosis. The controlled movements help you focus on form, making it a safe and accessible exercise.

Strategic Suggestions

Wall Angels can be an excellent addition to your routine for improving posture and supporting spinal health. Be consistent in performing them, and with time, you will likely notice improvements in your posture, shoulder strength, and upper back flexibility. Keep working on your form, and try to progressively challenge yourself by holding the position longer or increasing the range of motion. Remember, progress takes time, but with patience and consistency, Wall Angels can help you achieve a more aligned and stable posture, reducing discomfort and enhancing your overall well-being.

Scapular Squeezes for Shoulder Blade Strength

Scapular squeezes are a simple yet highly effective isometric exercise designed to strengthen the muscles around your shoulder blades (scapula) and upper back. For individuals with scoliosis, strengthening these muscles is crucial for improving posture and supporting the spine. The muscles around the shoulder blades help stabilize the upper back and prevent the rounding of the shoulders, which can often occur with scoliosis. This exercise also promotes better alignment, reduces neck and upper back tension, and encourages muscle balance, which can help alleviate discomfort associated with scoliosis.

What Are Scapular Squeezes and Why Are They Important?

Scapular squeezes are an exercise that targets the muscles between your shoulder blades, particularly the rhomboids and trapezius muscles. These muscles are responsible for keeping your shoulder blades in place and aiding in the movement of your arms and shoulders. When these muscles are weak, it can lead to poor posture, shoulder pain, and even increased tension in the neck and upper back.

For people with scoliosis, the muscles in the upper back, shoulders, and neck are often imbalanced. Some muscles may be overactive and tight, while others may be underactive and weak. Scapular squeezes can help to correct this imbalance by strengthening the muscles that support the shoulders and upper back, ultimately promoting better posture and reducing pain.

How to Perform Scapular Squeezes

To perform scapular squeezes correctly, follow these simple steps:

1. Start with Proper Posture

Stand or sit tall, ensuring that your back is straight and your shoulders are relaxed. Imagine a string attached to the top of your head, gently pulling you upwards to maintain an elongated spine. Your arms should be at your sides, with your elbows slightly bent.

2. Engage Your Core

Before beginning the movement, engage your core muscles. Gently draw your belly button toward your spine to help stabilize your torso. This will provide better support for your lower back and prevent any excessive arching during the exercise.

3. Squeeze Your Shoulder Blades Together

Slowly draw your shoulder blades together as if you're trying to pinch a pencil between them. Focus on moving from your shoulder blades, rather than your arms. Your elbows should remain relaxed, and your hands should stay by your sides. Make sure that the squeeze comes from the muscles between your shoulder blades, not from the arms or neck.

4. Hold the Squeeze

Once you've brought your shoulder blades together, hold the position for 5-10 seconds. Keep your chest open and your shoulders down. Avoid shrugging your shoulders up toward your ears.

5. Release and Repeat

Slowly release the squeeze and return to the starting position. Try to perform 10-15 repetitions, gradually increasing the hold time as your strength improves. Aim for 2-3 sets, and remember to breathe deeply throughout the exercise.

Modifications and Tips for Scapular Squeezes

While scapular squeezes are a simple exercise, there are several ways to modify them to match your current fitness level or to make them more challenging over time.

1. Start with Smaller Squeezes

If you're new to this exercise, it may be difficult to squeeze your shoulder blades fully together at first. That's okay—start with a smaller squeeze and gradually work on increasing the range of motion. With time, your strength and mobility will improve.

2. Add Resistance

Once you're comfortable with scapular squeezes, you can add resistance to make the exercise more challenging. One way to do this is by using a resistance band. Hold the band with both hands and stretch it as you perform the squeeze. This added resistance will help strengthen the muscles even more.

3. Perform in Different Positions

If you're finding it difficult to engage your shoulder blades while standing, try doing scapular squeezes while lying on your stomach or on your back. These positions can help you focus more on the shoulder blade muscles.

4. Mind the Shoulders

It's important not to shrug your shoulders while doing this exercise. Focus on keeping your shoulders down and away from your ears. This ensures that you're targeting the correct muscles—the ones between your shoulder blades—rather than the upper trapezius or neck muscles.

5. Use Visual Cues

To make the exercise more effective, visualize trying to bring your shoulder blades together as much as possible. Some people find it helpful to imagine that they're trying to hold a small ball between their shoulder blades.

Benefits of Scapular Squeezes for Scoliosis

Here are some of the key benefits:

1. Improved Posture

One of the primary benefits of scapular squeezes is improved posture. Strengthening the muscles around the shoulder blades helps pull the shoulders back, preventing the rounding that often occurs with scoliosis. As a result, this exercise can help create a more natural alignment of the spine and prevent further curvature.

2. Strengthened Upper Back Muscles:

Scapular squeezes target the muscles in the upper back, particularly the rhomboids and trapezius. These muscles are essential for stabilizing the shoulder blades and providing support to the spine. When these muscles are strong, they help keep the upper back in proper alignment, reducing strain on the spine.

3. Reduced Neck and Upper Back Tension

People with scoliosis often experience tension in the neck and upper back, especially in areas where muscle imbalances are present. Scapular squeezes help alleviate this tension by strengthening the muscles that support the shoulder blades and upper back, thereby reducing strain on the neck and spine.

4. Improved Shoulder Mobility

Scapular squeezes can also improve shoulder mobility. It is great for people with scoliosis, as restricted shoulder movement can affect the overall function and flexibility of the upper body.

5. Better Muscle Balance

Scoliosis can lead to muscle imbalances, where some muscles become overactive while others are underactive. Scapular squeezes help to correct these imbalances by strengthening the muscles of the upper back and shoulders.

6. Prevention of Further Spinal Misalignment

Strengthening the muscles of the upper back and shoulders can help prevent the progression of scoliosis by providing better support for the spine. The muscles act as a stabilizing force, reducing the risk of further misalignment and discomfort.

Strategic Suggestions

To get the most benefit from scapular squeezes, consistency is key. Perform them regularly, and as you build strength, try to gradually increase the hold time and the number of repetitions. If you're looking for additional challenge, incorporate resistance bands or try variations of the exercise. Over time, scapular squeezes will help improve your posture, strengthen your upper back, and reduce discomfort from scoliosis. As always, listen to your body, and avoid overexertion. Make scapular squeezes a part of your daily routine for long-lasting benefits.

Pelvic Tilts for Lower Back Support

Pelvic tilts are a fantastic isometric exercise for strengthening the muscles of your lower back, hips, and core, which are crucial areas of support for individuals with scoliosis. These muscles play an essential role in stabilizing the spine and preventing further misalignment, so it's important to keep them strong and engaged. Pelvic tilts target your pelvic region and lower back, helping to alleviate pain, reduce strain, and improve posture. For people with scoliosis, this exercise can provide significant relief by correcting pelvic tilt imbalances and promoting proper spinal alignment.

What Are Pelvic Tilts and Why Are They Important?

Pelvic tilts involve a small, controlled movement of your pelvis that helps engage the muscles of your lower back and abdomen. When you tilt your pelvis in different directions, you strengthen the muscles that support your spine, which can help reduce discomfort caused by scoliosis. The exercise is especially helpful for individuals with an exaggerated curve in the lower spine (lumbar region) or those who experience chronic lower back pain.

In scoliosis, the misalignment of the spine often causes imbalances in the muscles surrounding the pelvis and lower back. Weak muscles in these areas can make it difficult to maintain proper posture, leading to increased curvature and discomfort. Pelvic tilts help to address these imbalances by targeting key muscles that support the lower back and pelvic region.

How to Perform Pelvic Tilts

To perform pelvic tilts properly, follow these steps:

1. Get into Position

Lie on your back on a firm surface, such as a yoga mat or the floor. Bend your knees so that your feet are flat on the floor, with your legs hip-width apart. Keep your arms relaxed at your sides, palms facing down.

2. Engage Your Core

Gently tighten your abdominal muscles to engage your core. This will help protect your lower back and provide better support during the exercise. Imagine pulling your belly button toward your spine as you prepare to move your pelvis.

3. Tilt Your Pelvis

Slowly tilt your pelvis upward by gently pressing your lower back into the floor. This action should flatten the natural curve of your lower back, engaging your abdominal and gluteal muscles. At the same time, your pelvis should slightly shift upward as you flatten the lower back against the floor.

4. Hold the Position

Hold the pelvic tilt position for 5-10 seconds, ensuring that your core and glute muscles remain engaged. Breathe deeply and focus on keeping the movement controlled. Avoid arching your back or using momentum to complete the tilt—your muscles should do all the work.

5. Return to Starting Position

Slowly release the pelvic tilt and return to the starting position with a slight natural curve in your lower back. Take a deep breath and relax for a moment before repeating the movement.

6. Repeat

Perform 10-15 repetitions, aiming for 2-3 sets. Then, gradually increase the number of repetitions or hold the position for a longer period of time.

Modifications and Tips for Pelvic Tilts

While pelvic tilts are a simple exercise, there are several modifications and tips you can incorporate to make the exercise more effective or suited to your specific needs:

1. Start Slowly

If you're new to pelvic tilts, start by performing the movement slowly and gently. Focus on engaging your abdominal muscles and controlling the movement of your pelvis. As you gain strength, you can increase the speed and intensity.

2. Add Resistance

Once you're comfortable with pelvic tilts, you can increase the challenge by adding resistance. This can be done by placing a small weight, such as a sandbag or medicine ball, on your pelvis. As you tilt your pelvis upward, the added resistance will help further strengthen your core and lower back muscles.

3. Incorporate Breathing

Remember to breathe deeply and steadily throughout the exercise. Inhale as you prepare for the tilt and exhale as you engage your core and lift your pelvis. Breathing properly during this exercise can help maintain control and reduce tension in your muscles.

4. Focus on the Muscles

During pelvic tilts, it's important to focus on the muscles you're engaging. Visualize your lower back pressing into the floor and your pelvis tilting upward as you work the muscles of your core, glutes, and lower back. This will help ensure you are performing the exercise with proper form.

5. Modify for Lower Back Pain

If you experience pain in your lower back, make sure you're not arching or over-extending your spine while performing the tilt. If necessary, reduce the range of motion by performing smaller, more controlled tilts. You can also try placing a pillow under your knees for added support.

Benefits of Pelvic Tilts for Scoliosis

Here are some of the main benefits of pelvic tilts:

1. Improved Lower Back Support

Pelvic tilts strengthen the muscles in your lower back and core, which helps provide better support for your spine. This support is crucial for individuals with scoliosis, as it helps prevent further misalignment of the spine and alleviates discomfort.

2. Increased Spinal Stability

The exercise strengthens the muscles surrounding the spine, improving its stability and reducing the risk of injury. A stable spine is essential for individuals with scoliosis, as it helps prevent excessive curvature and keeps the body in proper alignment.

3. Pelvic Alignment

Pelvic tilts help correct imbalances in the pelvis, which can contribute to scoliosis-related pain and discomfort. When you improve pelvic alignment, the exercise promotes better spinal alignment overall, leading to a more even distribution of weight and reduced strain on the body.

4. Enhanced Posture

Pelvic tilts encourage better posture by strengthening the muscles that support the lower back and pelvis. As these muscles become stronger, your posture improves, reducing the tendency for the spine to curve unnaturally.

5. Alleviation of Lower Back Pain

For individuals with scoliosis, lower back pain is a common complaint. Pelvic tilts help alleviate this pain by strengthening the muscles that support the lower back and improving flexibility. The movement also helps release tension in the lower back and hips, providing relief from tightness and discomfort.

6. Core Strength

Pelvic tilts engage the muscles of your core, including your abdominal and glute muscles. Strengthening these muscles is essential for supporting the spine and preventing the development of muscle imbalances, which can exacerbate scoliosis.

Strategic Suggestions

Pelvic tilts are an excellent way to improve lower back support and address spinal imbalances related to scoliosis. However, to see the best results, it's important to stay consistent with your practice. Aim to incorporate pelvic tilts into your daily routine, gradually increasing the intensity as your strength improves. If you're unsure about your form, consider working with a physical therapist who can provide guidance and ensure that you're performing the exercise correctly. As you continue with pelvic tilts, you'll notice improvements in your posture, strength, and overall spinal health.

Chapter 7: Isometric Exercises for Daily Activities

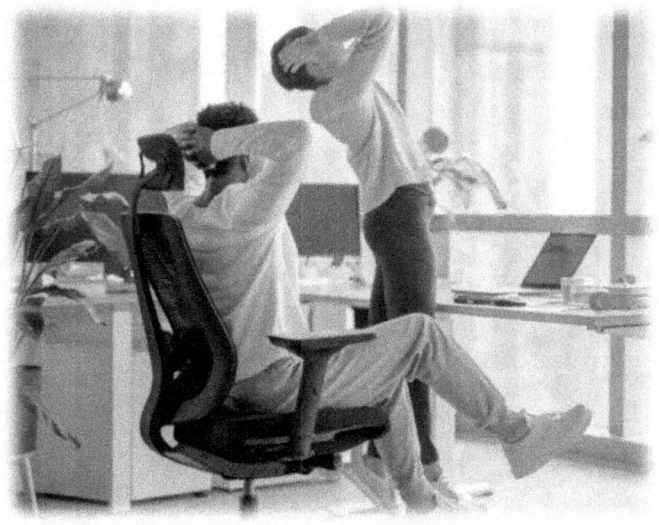

In today's world, many of us spend a significant amount of time sitting at desks or in front of computers, especially during work hours. While sitting itself isn't inherently bad, poor posture and lack of movement can lead to muscle imbalances, back pain, and even exacerbate scoliosis over time. A great way to counteract this is When you incorporate isometric exercises, such as chair sits, into your daily routine. These exercises are simple but effective in improving posture, strengthening your core muscles, and offering relief for your spine, all while you're seated.

Chair Sits for Office Workouts

Chair sits are isometric exercises that focus on engaging your core muscles, particularly the muscles of the lower back and abdomen, while seated. In this position, you perform a series of subtle movements designed to activate and strengthen key muscles without requiring any complex equipment or a change in posture. Chair sits are particularly beneficial for people with scoliosis who spend long hours sitting at a desk, as they help activate muscles that might otherwise remain inactive. They also promote spinal stability and posture control.

When we sit for extended periods, especially with poor posture, our spine becomes rounded or misaligned, and our muscles become weak and fatigued. Over time, this can lead to discomfort and potentially worsen spinal curves. Chair sits help you combat these issues by keeping your muscles engaged and supporting proper spinal alignment throughout the day.

How to Perform Chair Sits

Performing chair sits is simple and can be done at any time during your workday or even during a break, while waiting for something, or just as a reminder to engage your muscles. Here's how to perform this exercise properly:

1. Find a Good Chair

Start by sitting upright in a sturdy chair with your feet flat on the ground and your knees at a 90-degree angle. Your back should be straight, and your shoulders should be relaxed, not hunched. The goal is to maintain a neutral spine and avoid slouching.

2. Engage Your Core

Once you are sitting upright, gently tighten your abdominal muscles. Imagine pulling your belly button inward toward your spine. This engagement should be subtle but firm. Make sure to avoid holding your breath—deep breathing is key while performing this exercise.

3. Tilt Your Pelvis

To ensure you are working your core muscles, try gently tilting your pelvis slightly forward by pulling your hips into alignment with your torso. You should feel your lower back engaging as you tilt. This will help to activate the muscles in your abdomen and lower back, providing better support to your spine.

4. Hold the Position

Hold this engaged position for about 10-15 seconds. While holding the position, focus on keeping your back straight and maintaining a slight pelvic tilt. Avoid leaning forward or slouching—keep your posture tall and your core muscles engaged.

5. Release and Relax

After holding for a few seconds, slowly release the tension in your core and relax for a brief moment. It's essential to maintain control of the release, as this can help prevent any unnecessary strain on your muscles.

6. Repeat

Aim to perform 5-10 repetitions of the exercise, depending on how comfortable you feel. Over time, you can gradually increase the duration you hold the position or the number of repetitions as your strength improves.

Modifications and Tips for Chair Sits

If you find chair sits difficult or need to make adjustments to accommodate any discomfort or difficulty maintaining the position, here are some modifications and tips:

1. Start Slow

If you're new to this exercise, begin by holding the engaged position for just a few seconds. As you get used to the sensation of engaging your core, you can gradually increase the length of time you hold the contraction.

2. Use a Back Support

If your chair does not provide enough lumbar support, consider using a small cushion or lumbar roll behind your lower back to help you maintain a natural spinal curve. This can support your posture and make the exercise easier.

3. Focus on Breathing

While holding the position, be sure to breathe deeply. Inhale through your nose, allowing your lungs to fill with air, and exhale through your mouth. This helps maintain a relaxed state while still engaging your muscles.

4. Check Your Posture Regularly

Throughout your workday, remind yourself to check your posture and engage your core muscles regularly. Sitting with a rounded back or slouched posture can diminish the benefits of chair sits. Consider setting a timer to remind yourself to engage your core every 30 minutes.

5. Add Movement

Once you're comfortable with the basic chair sit, try incorporating slight variations. For example, try gently lifting one foot off the floor while maintaining your posture and core engagement, alternating legs. This small movement engages your hip flexors and adds a challenge to the exercise.

Benefits of Chair Sits for Scoliosis

Incorporating chair sits into your daily routine offers numerous benefits, especially if you spend long hours sitting. Here are the key advantages of performing this exercise regularly:

1. Improved Posture

Chair sits help to improve posture by strengthening the muscles that support your spine. As you maintain the engaged position, you reinforce the natural curvature of your spine, which is essential for those with scoliosis.

2. Core Strength

Engaging your core muscles while seated strengthens your abdomen and lower back, which are critical for spinal stability. A strong core supports proper posture and helps reduce discomfort associated with scoliosis.

3. Reduced Back Pain

Chair sits can reduce the risk of back pain, which is common for people with scoliosis. Strengthening these muscles can help relieve pressure on the spine and reduce discomfort.

4. Muscle Activation

Sitting for long periods can cause muscles to weaken, but chair sits activate key muscle groups that might otherwise remain inactive. When you engage your core, lower back, and pelvic muscles, you help maintain muscle tone and improve overall strength.

5. Improved Spinal Alignment

Maintaining a proper spinal alignment throughout the day is especially important for individuals with scoliosis. Chair sits help encourage this alignment by engaging the muscles that support the spine and helping to correct imbalances.

6. Prevention of Postural Deformities

Performing isometric exercises like chair sits helps prevent the development of postural deformities, such as slouching, which can worsen scoliosis. Regular engagement of your core and back muscles can keep your posture in check and prevent further misalignment.

Strategic Suggestions

To get the most out of chair sits, it's important to make this exercise a consistent part of your routine. Set reminders throughout your workday to engage your core and practice proper posture. Over time, you'll notice improved spinal stability and reduced back discomfort. As your strength improves, you can try adding variations or combining this exercise with other isometric movements to further enhance your core stability. Stay consistent, and soon enough, your body will thank you!

Isometric Walking Drills for Improved Balance

Balance is essential for maintaining proper posture, especially for individuals with scoliosis. When the spine is misaligned, balance can often become compromised, leading to discomfort, difficulty walking, or even falls. Isometric walking drills are a fantastic way to improve your balance and strengthen the muscles that help keep your body upright and stable. These exercises focus on engaging various muscle groups in the lower body and core while holding a still position during walking motions, offering both strength and stability benefits.

What Are Isometric Walking Drills and Why Are They Important?

Isometric walking drills combine the principles of isometric exercises with walking movements to enhance stability, proprioception (your sense of body position), and coordination. In these drills, you hold certain positions while engaging your core and lower body muscles, providing a way to build balance without moving too quickly or requiring high-impact activity. These drills activate muscles that help stabilize your spine and maintain proper posture while walking.

People with scoliosis often struggle with maintaining balance due to an uneven weight distribution across the spine and trunk. These isometric walking drills target your posture and core muscles, reinforcing your body's ability to stay centered and aligned while walking or performing daily activities.

How to Perform Isometric Walking Drills

1. Start in a Neutral Position

Begin by standing tall with your feet hip-width apart, ensuring that your body weight is evenly distributed. Your knees should be slightly bent, and your shoulders should be relaxed and aligned with your hips. Stand tall, with your spine straight and your chin parallel to the ground.

2. Engage Your Core

Before you begin the walking drill, take a moment to engage your core muscles. Gently tighten your abdominal muscles, pulling your belly button toward your spine. This will provide stability to your torso and protect your lower back while performing the exercise. Focus on keeping your core engaged throughout the drill.

3. Lift One Leg

Begin by lifting one leg to a 90-degree angle at the hip. The knee should be bent, with your foot hovering just above the ground. Hold this position for 10-15 seconds, making sure your core stays engaged and your posture remains upright. You should feel the muscles in your hip, glutes, and core activating as you hold this stance.

4. Hold and Balance

While holding the leg up, focus on maintaining balance. Avoid leaning to one side or overcompensating with your upper body. Ensure that your standing leg is slightly bent to help you stabilize. If you need extra support, use a wall or chair nearby to assist you, but try to rely mostly on your muscles for stability.

5. Switch Legs

After holding the first leg up for the prescribed amount of time, slowly lower it and lift the opposite leg. Repeat the same movement, engaging the core, holding the position, and maintaining balance. The key here is to focus on stability and control rather than speed. Aim for 10-15 seconds on each leg.

6. Add Walking Movements (Optional)

Once you're comfortable with the basic isometric hold, you can incorporate a more dynamic movement. Start by walking forward in small, controlled steps, ensuring that you maintain your balance and posture. As you take each step, engage your core muscles, keeping your spine aligned. With practice, your body will begin to naturally engage these muscles with each step, improving your balance while walking.

7. Repeat the Drills

Try to perform the isometric walking drills for about 10-15 minutes daily. You can increase the duration of each hold as your strength improves. Aim for a total of 5-10 repetitions for each leg. Consistency is key in building muscle memory and improving your balance over time.

Modifications and Tips for Isometric Walking Drills

If you're new to isometric walking drills or need modifications to make the exercise more comfortable, here are some helpful tips:

1. Use a Supportive Surface

If balancing is challenging, practice near a stable surface such as a chair, table, or wall. This will help you feel more secure while learning the proper technique. As you gain confidence, try to perform the drill without holding onto anything.

2. Start Slow

Begin with short holds (5-10 seconds) and work your way up. Holding each leg up for an extended period can be difficult, so it's important to start at a level where you feel comfortable and gradually increase the time as your strength and balance improve.

3. Engage Your Glutes and Hips

Focus on engaging your glute muscles and hip flexors as you hold each leg up. These muscles are critical for maintaining stability and controlling your balance. Squeeze your glutes as if you're trying to push your pelvis forward slightly to create better alignment and support.

4. Use a Mirror

If possible, practice in front of a mirror to check your posture. Make sure your back is straight, your shoulders are aligned with your hips, and your chest is lifted. Keeping your body aligned will improve the effectiveness of the drill and prevent any compensatory movements.

5. Increase Intensity Gradually

As you become more confident in the drill, challenge yourself by holding each position for longer durations or incorporating small steps between holds. You can also practice this exercise on a balance pad or soft surface to increase the challenge.

Benefits of Isometric Walking Drills for Scoliosis

Isometric walking drills offer numerous benefits for people with scoliosis, particularly when it comes to improving balance, posture, and spinal alignment. Here are some of the key advantages:

1. Improved Balance

These drills target the muscles responsible for maintaining balance, particularly in the core and lower body. When you consistently engage these muscles, you can enhance your ability to stay upright and prevent falls, which is especially important for individuals with scoliosis who may experience balance issues.

2. Stronger Core Muscles

Engaging your core during these drills strengthens the muscles that support your spine, reducing strain on the back and helping to improve posture. A stronger core also helps to alleviate discomfort and prevent further curvature progression.

3. Enhanced Spinal Stability

Isometric walking drills help stabilize the spine by improving posture and engaging muscles that support the trunk and hips. This is important for scoliosis patients, as it can reduce the risk of further spinal misalignment.

4. Better Posture

As you practice maintaining balance with proper posture, you'll notice improvements in your overall alignment. Consistently holding these isometric positions helps reinforce the correct posture and supports spinal health.

5. Reduced Back Pain

Strengthening the muscles surrounding your spine can help alleviate the pressure that causes discomfort in the lower back. With stronger and more engaged muscles, you may experience relief from the chronic pain often associated with scoliosis.

Strategic Suggestions

To gain the full benefits from isometric walking drills, consistency is key. Incorporate these exercises into your daily routine, even if just for a few minutes. Over time, you'll notice improvements in your balance, posture, and overall stability. Additionally, as you build strength in your core and lower body, these exercises will help to reduce discomfort and enhance your ability to perform other daily activities. Keep practicing, and soon you'll see noticeable progress in your balance and posture!

Core Engagement While Standing

Core engagement is essential for maintaining good posture, spinal health, and overall balance. While many exercises emphasize core strengthening in lying or sitting positions, it's crucial to remember that your core is just as active when you're standing. For individuals with scoliosis, core engagement while standing can significantly improve posture, reduce strain on the back, and help prevent further spinal curvature. In this section, we'll explore how to properly engage your core while standing, the benefits of doing so, and how to incorporate this practice into your daily routine.

What Is Core Engagement While Standing?

Core engagement while standing refers to activating the muscles of your abdomen, lower back, and pelvis to maintain stability and proper posture while on your feet. When your core is engaged, your spine is more aligned, and the muscles surrounding it provide better support. For individuals with scoliosis, this is especially important because it helps correct imbalances, reduces pain, and promotes a more neutral spine position.

Core engagement is not just about tightening your abs; it involves activating the muscles that support your entire trunk. The core includes muscles such as the rectus abdominis (the "six-pack" muscles), the obliques (muscles along the sides of your abdomen), the transversus abdominis (deep abdominal muscles), and the muscles in your lower back and pelvic floor. Engaging these muscles effectively can stabilize your spine, improve posture, and reduce discomfort.

How to Properly Engage Your Core While Standing

Here's a step-by-step guide on how to properly activate your core muscles and maintain a stable, aligned posture:

1. Start in a Neutral Standing Position

Stand tall with your feet hip-width apart. Your weight should be evenly distributed between both feet, and your knees should be slightly bent. Avoid locking your knees or leaning forward or backward. Make sure your pelvis is in a neutral position, not tilted forward or backward.

2. Check Your Posture

Stand with your shoulders relaxed but not slumped. Your ears should be aligned with your shoulders, your shoulders aligned with your hips, and your hips aligned with your ankles. This alignment creates a straight line from your head to your feet, which is essential for good posture.

3. Engage Your Lower Abs

To engage your core, gently pull your belly button toward your spine. This action activates the deep muscles of your abdomen, including the transversus abdominis. It should feel like you're bracing your abdomen without holding your breath. Think of it as preparing your body for a gentle punch to the stomach — firm but relaxed.

4. Activate Your Glutes and Lower Back

Along with your abdominal muscles, engage your glutes and the muscles in your lower back. Squeeze your glutes as if you're trying to tighten your waistband. This helps stabilize your pelvis and supports your lower back. Additionally, gently lengthen your lower back muscles by imagining your spine growing taller.

5. Maintain Breathing

One of the key aspects of core engagement is maintaining normal breathing. As you engage your core, remember not to hold your breath. Take slow, deep breaths in and out while keeping your core muscles engaged. This ensures that you're not overexerting yourself, and it helps your body remain balanced and relaxed.

6. Hold the Engagement

Once you've activated your core, hold the position. It's not necessary to keep your core tight all the time, but you should aim to engage it whenever you're standing for extended periods or performing tasks like walking, lifting, or even doing household chores.

7. Correct Posture Check

While engaging your core, regularly check your posture to ensure that you're not slouching or leaning too far in one direction. A common mistake is to overcompensate and arch your lower back too much, which can create more discomfort. Keep your spine in neutral alignment, avoiding excessive curvature.

8. Practice Regularly

Initially, you may need to remind yourself to engage your core while standing. With practice, it will become a natural part of your posture, allowing you to maintain a stable and balanced position throughout the day.

Benefits of Core Engagement While Standing for Scoliosis

For individuals with scoliosis, engaging your core while standing offers several benefits that can help manage symptoms, prevent pain, and improve overall function. Here are some of the key advantages:

1. Improved Posture

Engaging your core helps you maintain a more upright and aligned posture. This is crucial for individuals with scoliosis, as it can prevent further spinal curvature and reduce the risk of discomfort or muscle imbalances caused by poor posture.

2. Reduced Back Pain

Strengthening your core muscles can alleviate pressure on your spine and reduce the strain on your back. A strong core helps distribute your weight more evenly and keeps the spine in a more neutral position, relieving pain that might otherwise result from scoliosis-related imbalances.

3. Spinal Stability

By engaging the core muscles, you provide better support to your spine. This stability helps protect against further misalignment and reduces the risk of injury while performing daily activities.

4. Increased Balance

Engaging the core also enhances your overall balance. When you activate the muscles that control your trunk and pelvis, you improve your ability to stand and move with more control. This can reduce the risk of falls, especially if scoliosis affects your balance or coordination.

5. Enhanced Muscle Coordination

Core engagement strengthens the muscles that support your posture, improving the coordination between the muscles in your back, abdomen, and pelvis. This leads to more efficient movement patterns and a reduction in compensatory postures that can worsen scoliosis.

Modifications and Tips for Core Engagement While Standing

If you're new to core engagement or find it challenging to maintain for long periods, here are some modifications and tips that can help you get the most out of this practice:

1. Use a Mirror

Practice in front of a mirror to check your posture and alignment. This visual feedback will help you ensure that your spine is neutral, and your shoulders, hips, and ankles are aligned.

2. Start with Short Intervals

If you find it difficult to engage your core for long periods, start by holding the engagement for short intervals, such as 15-30 seconds.

Gradually increase the time as your core strength improves.

3. Incorporate Movement

While standing, incorporate small movements like shifting your weight from one foot to the other, bending your knees slightly, or gently swaying your hips. These movements will help reinforce the core engagement and prevent stiffness from holding a position for too long.

4. Take Breaks

If you're standing for long periods, make sure to take breaks and rest. Stand up, stretch, or walk around to give your muscles a break. This will prevent fatigue and help maintain optimal posture.

5. Practice While Doing Daily Tasks

Engage your core while standing during daily activities, such as brushing your teeth, waiting for the bus, or doing dishes. The more you practice, the more natural it will become to maintain core engagement throughout the day.

Strategic Suggestions

Incorporating core engagement into your standing posture is a simple but effective way to improve spinal health, balance, and overall comfort for individuals with scoliosis. Stay consistent with this practice, and over time, you'll notice improvements in your posture, reduced back pain, and enhanced stability. When you strengthen the muscles that support your spine and trunk, you'll create a more stable foundation for all of your daily activities. Keep practicing, and remember to be patient with your progress.

Chapter 8: Safety and Progression in Isometric Exercises

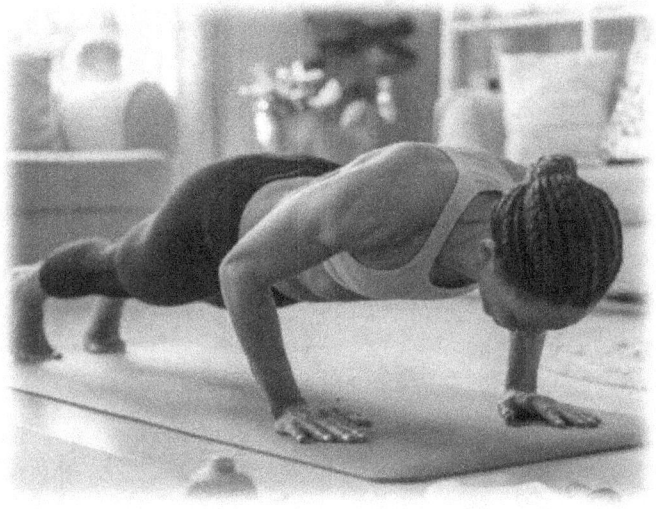

When beginning any new exercise, especially with scoliosis, it's essential to approach it with caution and patience. Isometric exercises, in particular, can be very effective for strengthening the muscles that support your spine, but they need to be introduced slowly and progressively. If you push yourself too hard at the start, you risk overexerting muscles or worsening discomfort. In this section, we'll explore how to safely begin with short holds and gradually increase the intensity and duration of your isometric exercises.

Starting with Short Holds and Gradual Increases

Starting with short holds allows you to ease into the routine of isometric exercises without overwhelming your muscles or joints. It's all about building a solid foundation. Just like when you're learning a new skill, you wouldn't rush the process. Starting small helps your body adjust to the new movements and allows you to focus on proper form.

For someone with scoliosis, engaging in isometric exercises requires a careful balance. Your muscles might be used to compensating for spinal imbalances, and placing too much strain on them too soon can lead to discomfort or injury. Short holds give your body the time it needs to adapt, while you also learn how to engage the correct muscles without overworking them.

How to Start with Short Holds

1. Choose a Simple Exercise

Begin with basic isometric exercises that don't require too much physical demand but still provide the benefits you need. For instance, a simple wall sit or plank hold can work wonders for your core strength without being too intense. The key is to pick exercises that target your core and back muscles, as these are often the areas that need the most support when managing scoliosis.

2. Start with 10-15 Second Holds

If you're new to isometric exercises, start by holding a position for just 10 to 15 seconds. This is long enough to activate the muscles and give you a sense of how your body responds. It's also short enough to ensure that you won't feel overexerted. The first time you try, you might only hold for 5-10 seconds, which is perfectly fine.

3. Focus on Proper Form

Ensure that you maintain the correct posture while holding each position. For example, if you're doing a wall sit, make sure your knees are directly above your ankles, and your back is straight. Engaging the right muscles is key, especially for scoliosis, where muscle imbalances are common.

4. Breathe Deeply and Regularly

Don't hold your breath during isometric holds. It's tempting to hold your breath when you feel the strain, but this can cause unnecessary tension. Instead, focus on slow, deep breathing as you hold the position. This helps relax your muscles and ensures you're not over-stressing your body.

5. Rest and Recover

After each short hold, rest for at least 30 seconds to a minute before attempting another set. Use this time to relax your muscles and regain your strength. Starting with short holds means you're less likely to experience fatigue or strain, so enjoy the rest period to reset.

6. Pay Attention to Discomfort

While some muscle tension is expected when doing isometric exercises, discomfort or pain is not. If you feel any sharp pain or discomfort, stop the exercise immediately. Your body may need more time to adjust, or you might need to tweak your form. It's always better to be cautious and make sure you're not pushing too hard.

7. Gradually Increasing Holds

Once you feel comfortable with the shorter holds and have practiced good form consistently, you can start to increase the duration of each hold. Gradually increasing the hold time helps you build strength without overwhelming your muscles.

8. Increase Duration by 5 Seconds

After a week or two of practicing 10-15 second holds, you can begin to increase your hold times by 5 seconds each time. For example, you can move from holding a plank for 15 seconds to 20 seconds. Don't rush the progression — it's important to allow your muscles and joints to adapt. Every person's progress will be different, so don't compare your timeline to others.

9. Increase Hold Times for One Set

Instead of increasing the number of sets, try increasing the hold time for a single set first. For instance, instead of doing two 15-second wall sits, you can challenge yourself to hold one wall sit for 20-30 seconds. Once you feel confident with this, you can increase the number of sets as well.

10. Listen to Your Body

As you increase your hold times, continue to listen to your body. If you notice any pain or discomfort, take a break and decrease your hold time. Remember, progression is not about pushing yourself to the limit, but rather about building strength over time. Your body will tell you when it's ready to handle more.

11. Use a Timer

To keep track of your progress, use a timer or stopwatch. This helps you stay on target with your progression and ensures that you're gradually increasing your holds. It also takes away the guesswork and allows you to focus on the exercise itself.

12. Alternate Exercises for Balanced Progression

If you're starting to feel that one exercise is getting easier, it's a good idea to alternate between different isometric exercises. This will help target various muscle groups and prevent overuse injuries. For example, alternate between planks, wall sits, and side planks, ensuring a full-body approach to strengthening.

Benefits of Gradual Progression

Starting with short holds and gradually increasing them offers several benefits, especially for individuals managing scoliosis. When you pace yourself, you avoid the risk of injury, prevent muscle strain, and ensure steady improvement over time. Gradual progression also helps you develop consistency, which is key for long-term success.

In the context of scoliosis, gradual progression supports your body's need for balance. Since scoliosis can cause muscle imbalances, progressing slowly gives your muscles time to strengthen evenly and support the spine more effectively.

Strategic Suggestions

Remember, slow and steady wins the race. As you begin with short holds and increase them gradually, consistency is key. Track your progress regularly to ensure you're staying on the right track. This will not only help you see physical improvements, but it will also give you the motivation to continue. Be patient, listen to your body, and enjoy the process of building strength at a pace that works for you.

Recognizing and Avoiding Painful Movements

When engaging in isometric exercises, especially if you're managing scoliosis, it's vital to distinguish between the normal muscle tension that comes with strengthening and any pain that signals potential harm. Pain is your body's way of telling you something is wrong, and while some discomfort may be expected when working on muscle endurance, it is crucial to avoid pushing your body beyond its limits. In this section, we'll discuss how to recognize and avoid painful movements during isometric exercises, ensuring that your practice remains safe and effective.

Understanding the Difference Between Discomfort and Pain

Before you can avoid painful movements, it's important to understand the difference between discomfort and pain. During isometric exercises, you'll likely feel some level of discomfort as your muscles work hard to maintain a specific position. This is natural and is a sign that your muscles are being activated. However, pain is a sharp, often sudden sensation that can be felt in the muscles, joints, or bones. Pain may also radiate to other areas of the body, and it can feel like a burning or stabbing sensation.

Discomfort, on the other hand, is typically a mild to moderate ache that you can push through, knowing that it's part of the strengthening process.

Recognizing Pain During Isometric Exercises

During isometric exercises, you may experience a variety of sensations in your body. While some level of muscle fatigue is normal, pain is a red flag that should not be ignored. Here are common signs that you might be experiencing pain rather than normal discomfort:

1. Sharp or Stabbing Pain

If you feel a sudden sharp or stabbing pain, it's a clear signal that something isn't right. This type of pain may come from your joints, muscles, or even your spine, especially if you have scoliosis. Always stop immediately if you experience this type of pain, as it could indicate strain, sprain, or other injuries.

2. Radiating Pain

Sometimes, pain may not stay in one spot. If the pain starts in one area and radiates to others (for example, pain in your lower back radiating to your hips or legs), it's a warning sign that you might be overexerting yourself or not maintaining proper form. This could also indicate a deeper issue, such as nerve irritation or muscle strain.

3. Numbness or Tingling

Numbness or a tingling sensation in your arms, legs, or back is a warning sign that your nerves may be involved. This type of pain requires immediate attention, as it could be a sign of nerve compression or other issues that need medical attention.

4. Joint Pain

If you feel discomfort in your joints (such as knees, elbows, or wrists), this is often a sign that you're placing too much pressure on those areas during the exercise. Joint pain can be particularly concerning, as it can lead to inflammation or injury over time if not addressed properly.

5. Pain that Doesn't Go Away

If you notice that pain continues after you stop the exercise, or if it lasts for hours or days, it's a signal that something went wrong. Unlike muscle fatigue or soreness, which tends to subside after rest, lingering pain often indicates that the body has been overstrained.

Common Mistakes That Lead to Pain

Certain common mistakes in isometric exercises can lead to pain, especially for people with scoliosis who may already have muscle imbalances. Let's take a look at some of these mistakes and how you can avoid them.

1. Incorrect Posture

One of the most common causes of pain during isometric exercises is improper posture. When performing a wall sit, plank, or other exercises, maintaining correct body alignment is crucial. If your back is not aligned properly, it can put undue stress on your spine, leading to discomfort or pain. Always ensure your shoulders, hips, and knees are aligned and that you're engaging your core muscles to protect your lower back.

2. Overdoing the Exercise

Trying to hold a position for too long, or performing too many sets, can lead to muscle fatigue that turns into pain. It's essential to start with shorter holds and gradually increase the duration as your muscles adapt. Pushing too hard can strain the muscles or joints, which is especially problematic if you have scoliosis, as the body is already working harder to maintain proper alignment.

3. Sudden, Jerky Movements

Isometric exercises are meant to be slow and controlled. If you move too quickly or try to adjust your position too rapidly, you risk injuring yourself. For example, if you're holding a plank and suddenly shift your weight or change your position too quickly, you could strain your muscles. Always move with intention and control, focusing on slow, deliberate movements.

4. Not Engaging the Core

The core muscles are essential for maintaining stability, especially when performing isometric exercises. If you fail to engage your core during exercises like wall sits or planks, you might overcompensate by relying on other muscles, which could lead to pain in your back or neck. Always make sure you're engaging your core and keeping your spine in a neutral position.

How to Avoid Pain During Isometric Exercises

Now that you know how to recognize pain, here are some practical tips for avoiding it during your isometric exercise routine.

1. Warm Up Properly

Before starting your isometric exercises, always warm up with some gentle stretching and mobility exercises. A good warm-up prepares your muscles for the work ahead and helps prevent strains or sprains. Focus on areas that are most involved, like your back, hips, and legs, and gently stretch these areas to improve flexibility.

2. Start Slow and Build Gradually

It's tempting to push yourself to do more, but the key to avoiding pain is to start slow. Begin with short holds and gradually increase the duration and intensity over time. This will help your muscles and joints adapt without overloading them.

3. Focus on Form

Proper form is crucial when performing any exercise, and even more so with scoliosis. Always ensure you are maintaining the correct posture throughout each movement. If you're unsure, try recording yourself or asking a physical therapist for feedback.

4. Rest Between Sets

Don't skip your rest periods between sets, as isometric exercises are intense, and your muscles need time to recover.

5. Listen to Your Body

Above all, listen to your body. If something doesn't feel right, stop immediately. Adjust your form or take a break. Remember, there's no rush in building strength, and it's more important to progress safely than to push through pain.

Strategic Suggestions

If you find that pain persists or if you're unsure about your form, don't hesitate to consult a healthcare professional or a physical therapist. They can provide valuable guidance tailored to your specific needs and ensure that you're on the right track. When you focus on proper form, listening to your body, and progressing gradually, you can avoid painful movements and enjoy the benefits of isometric exercises for scoliosis.

Tracking Progress for Motivation

Tracking your progress in any exercise routine is key to staying motivated and ensuring that you're on the right path. This is especially true for isometric exercises, which can sometimes feel slow and subtle in terms of progress. When managing scoliosis, where the body might require extra support and stability, monitoring your progress can help you stay on track, measure improvements, and celebrate small victories along the way. In this section, we will discuss various ways to track your progress, how this can help you stay motivated, and why it is essential for your overall success.

Why Tracking Progress Matters

Tracking progress serves multiple purposes. First, it provides a clear picture of how far you've come, even when the results aren't immediately visible. It can be easy to feel discouraged if you're not seeing drastic changes in your body, but keeping track of subtle improvements can help you stay motivated. Progress doesn't always mean visible changes; it can also mean improved endurance, better form, or feeling more stable during exercises.

Secondly, tracking progress helps you avoid plateaus. Isometric exercises, while effective, can sometimes feel like they're not yielding immediate results. However, when you track your progress, you'll notice when it's time to increase the intensity or duration of your holds to challenge your muscles further. Without tracking, it's easy to get stuck in a routine that's too easy, causing a stall in improvement.

Finally, tracking your progress reinforces positive behaviors. When you see improvements, no matter how small, it boosts your confidence and makes you feel accomplished. This sense of achievement helps build motivation, making you more likely to stick with your exercise routine over the long term.

Methods of Tracking Progress

There are several ways to track your progress when doing isometric exercises for scoliosis. The goal is to find a method that is realistic and easy for you to maintain. Here are a few practical suggestions:

1. Recording Hold Duration

One of the most straightforward ways to track your progress is by noting how long you can hold each isometric exercise. For example, if you start with a wall sit and can only hold it for 15 seconds, aim to gradually increase that time by a few seconds each week. Keep a simple log where you record how long you can hold each position. Over time, you will see that your endurance is improving, which is a significant indicator of progress.

Tip: Try setting mini-goals. If you hold your position for 30 seconds one day, aim for 35 seconds in a few days, and continue building on that. Small, incremental increases help prevent burnout and keep you motivated.

2. Form Improvement Checklist

Isometric exercises, especially for scoliosis, rely heavily on proper form to prevent injury and ensure maximum effectiveness. Tracking the quality of your form is just as important as tracking time or repetitions. For each exercise, create a checklist of key posture points (like neutral spine position or engaged core) and rate your form at the end of each session. Over time, you'll notice that you need fewer reminders to maintain proper form.

Tip: Take photos or videos of your exercises to visually compare your form over time. This can be motivating as you start to see physical improvements in how you move.

3. Pain-Free Progress

Tracking your progress isn't just about building strength; it's also about improving the way your body feels during and after the exercises. If you experience discomfort or pain at the start, try tracking when you feel pain, how intense it is, and if it subsides with consistent practice. Over time, you should notice fewer or less intense pain episodes as your muscles and joints adapt. Recording these changes can give you positive reinforcement.

Tip: Keep a pain journal where you note the type of pain, its location, and its intensity. If you notice that certain exercises consistently cause pain, this can signal the need to adjust your form or try different variations of the exercise.

4. Tracking Muscle Fatigue

Another way to measure your progress is by noting how quickly your muscles fatigue. When you begin, you may feel tired after holding a plank for just a few seconds, but over time, you'll find that your muscles can endure the tension for longer periods without feeling fatigued. Tracking muscle fatigue is a great way to see your stamina increase.

Tip: Record how your muscles feel immediately after each set (i.e., how fatigued they are) and how long it takes them to recover. You'll notice that recovery time shortens as your strength builds.

5. Set Long-Term and Short-Term Goals

Setting both short-term and long-term goals for your isometric exercises gives you something tangible to work toward. Short-term goals could be as simple as increasing your hold time by 5 seconds in one week, while long-term goals could include reaching a specific duration or mastering a particular variation of an exercise. Review these goals regularly to stay focused and motivated.

Tip: Write down your goals and put them somewhere visible (like on a fridge or a mirror). When you meet them, celebrate your success and set a new goal.

Using Progress to Stay Motivated

Tracking your progress is only beneficial if you use that information to fuel your motivation. Here are some strategies for leveraging the progress you've tracked to stay inspired:

1. Celebrate Milestones

Each time you reach a new milestone, such as holding a plank for an extra 10 seconds or feeling less discomfort during wall sits, celebrate it! This could mean treating yourself to a healthy snack, a relaxing bath, or just taking a moment to reflect on how far you've come.

2. Reflect on Your Successes

It's easy to get discouraged if you focus only on the challenges ahead. Instead, take time to look back at how much progress you've made.

Reflecting on your successes reminds you that the hard work is paying off.

3. Adjust Goals Based on Progress

As you track your progress, you may find that your initial goals need to be adjusted. Maybe you're holding a plank longer than expected, or perhaps you've noticed significant improvement in muscle stability. Don't be afraid to raise the bar when you're ready. Adjusting your goals based on progress keeps you engaged and provides new challenges to work toward.

4. Stay Consistent

The key to continued progress is consistency. It's tempting to skip a session here and there, but keeping track of your progress makes it easier to stay on track. When you see the improvements you've made, you're more likely to stay consistent in your effort.

Strategic Suggestions

Tracking your progress is a powerful way to stay motivated, but remember that it's only one part of the puzzle. Keep challenging yourself with new goals, and celebrate each milestone along the way. Your progress will continue to build, and as your body strengthens, so will your confidence. Stay committed to the process, and you'll continue to see improvements that help you manage scoliosis and improve your overall health.

Chapter 9: Nutrition to Support Scoliosis Management

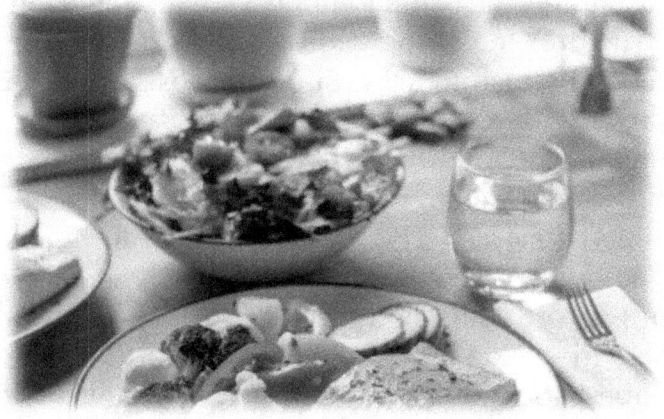

When managing scoliosis, supporting your bones is crucial to maintaining strength and flexibility, especially since your spine plays a key role in your body's alignment and overall well-being. Nutrients like calcium and vitamin D are essential for healthy bones, helping you strengthen and protect your spine as you work through isometric exercises and other treatments. Understanding these nutrients and how to incorporate them into your daily routine is a great first step toward supporting your scoliosis management.

Bone-Strengthening Nutrients: Calcium and Vitamin D

Calcium is the primary mineral that builds bone structure, ensuring bones stay strong and resistant to fractures. Since scoliosis can alter the alignment of the spine, it's even more important for those with scoliosis to have sufficient calcium intake to support bone health and reduce any risk of further complications. The bones in your spine, particularly, bear the brunt of your body's weight and physical activities. Adequate calcium ensures that these bones remain dense and strong enough to support your body's movements and help with overall spinal stability.

Vitamin D works alongside calcium to ensure it is absorbed properly into the bones. Without sufficient vitamin D, your body can't absorb calcium efficiently, which can lead to weaker bones over time.

Calcium-Rich Foods You Can Include in Your Diet

To support your spine, aim for calcium-rich foods that will help build and maintain strong bones. Some excellent sources of calcium include:

1. **Dairy Products**

Milk, cheese, and yogurt are some of the best sources of calcium. If you're lactose intolerant, lactose-free dairy products are available or you can choose plant-based options like almond or soy milk fortified with calcium.

2. **Leafy Green Vegetables**

Kale, spinach, and broccoli are not only packed with calcium but also full of other vitamins and minerals that support bone health.

3. **Fortified Foods**

Many products, like orange juice, cereals, and plant-based milks, are fortified with calcium to help you reach your daily intake if natural sources are limited.

4. **Tofu and Tempeh**

These soy products are high in calcium, making them a great choice for vegetarians and vegans.

Incorporating these foods into your meals will help you meet your daily calcium needs and contribute to stronger bones over time. Depending on your age, lifestyle, and health, you may need more or less calcium, so it's always wise to consult with your doctor to determine the exact amount for your situation.

Vitamin D: A Vital Partner for Calcium Absorption

Vitamin D is another critical nutrient that supports bone health by helping your body absorb calcium. While calcium builds your bones, vitamin D ensures that your bones can actually use the calcium effectively. Without vitamin D, you might consume calcium, but your body will not be able to absorb it properly, which could leave you with weaker bones over time.

Sun exposure is one of the best natural sources of vitamin D. Spending time outdoors, especially in the sun, helps your skin produce vitamin D naturally. However, it's important to balance sun exposure with skin safety. Too much sun can lead to skin damage or increase the risk of skin cancer, so use sunscreen or wear protective clothing while getting sun exposure.

In addition to sunlight, vitamin D is also found in various foods. Some of the best sources of vitamin D include:

- **Fatty Fish:** Salmon, mackerel, and sardines are excellent sources of vitamin D, as well as omega-3 fatty acids, which help reduce inflammation in the body.
- **Egg Yolks:** Eggs contain vitamin D, and the yolk is where it's found, so make sure

to include the whole egg in your diet if possible.
- **Fortified Foods:** Similar to calcium, many foods like milk, orange juice, and cereals are fortified with vitamin D to help people meet their daily requirements.
- **Mushrooms:** Certain varieties of mushrooms, like maitake and shiitake, contain vitamin D, particularly when exposed to sunlight during their growth process.

Getting enough vitamin D ensures that your body can absorb the calcium you're consuming, which is critical for maintaining bone health and supporting scoliosis management.

Balancing Calcium and Vitamin D for Optimal Bone Health

It's essential to get the right balance of calcium and vitamin D. Without enough vitamin D, your body might not absorb all the calcium you eat, even if you're consuming enough. Similarly, without adequate calcium, your bones will lack the strength needed to support your spine properly, even with plenty of vitamin D. If you're unsure about your levels, a blood test can provide insight into your specific needs, such as changes to your diet or take supplements.

For people with scoliosis, proper bone health is even more critical, as your spine's alignment needs extra support. A balanced intake of both calcium and vitamin D will help you reduce the risk of further complications and aid in building a strong foundation for exercises like isometric movements.

Strategic Suggestions

Ensuring that you're getting enough calcium and vitamin D is a simple yet powerful way to support your scoliosis management. Together, these nutrients will help keep your bones strong, improve calcium absorption, and support the isometric exercises you're incorporating into your routine. Stay mindful of your diet and make adjustments as needed to ensure you're giving your body what it needs to thrive.

Muscle-Supportive Nutrients: Protein, Magnesium, and Potassium

When managing scoliosis, muscle strength plays a vital role in supporting your spine. While we often focus on bones, your muscles are just as important for holding everything in place. Nutrients like protein, magnesium, and potassium are essential for muscle function and recovery. These nutrients work together to support muscle contraction, reduce cramping, and maintain overall muscle health. Understanding how to incorporate these nutrients into your diet can make a significant difference in the way your muscles feel and function, especially when combined with your isometric exercises for scoliosis.

Protein: The Building Block for Muscle Repair

Protein is the fundamental building block of muscle tissue. Your body uses it to repair and rebuild muscle fibers after physical activity. For those with scoliosis, strong and healthy muscles are essential for supporting the spine and improving posture. When you engage in exercises like isometric holds, your muscles are working to maintain a contracted position for a period of time. This can cause minor tears in muscle fibers, and protein helps repair these fibers, making them stronger over time.

To support your muscle recovery and strength, aim to include a variety of protein sources in your diet. Some excellent sources of protein include:

- **Lean Meats:** Chicken, turkey, and lean cuts of beef or pork are high in protein and can help with muscle repair and strength building.
- **Fish:** Salmon, tuna, and other fatty fish are packed with protein and also contain healthy omega-3 fatty acids, which help reduce muscle inflammation and support recovery.
- **Legumes:** Beans, lentils, and chickpeas are excellent plant-based sources of protein. They are also high in fiber, which helps with digestion.
- **Nuts and Seeds:** Almonds, sunflower seeds, chia seeds, and other nuts are rich in protein and healthy fats that support muscle health.
- **Dairy:** Milk, yogurt, and cheese provide both protein and calcium, making them great for muscle and bone support.

For optimal results, aim for a balanced intake of protein throughout the day. Try to incorporate protein into every meal, as your body requires a steady supply of this nutrient for muscle recovery and growth.

Magnesium: A Crucial Mineral for Muscle Function

Magnesium plays a key role in muscle function, including contraction and relaxation. It also helps to prevent muscle cramps, which can be particularly bothersome when engaging in physical activity, including exercises designed to help with scoliosis. When magnesium levels are low, you may experience muscle twitches, cramps, or spasms, which can interfere with your workouts and daily activities.

Magnesium also supports energy production and is involved in over 300 biochemical reactions in the body. For individuals with scoliosis, maintaining proper magnesium levels ensures that your muscles have the energy they need to stabilize your spine and support correct posture.

Some magnesium-rich foods to include in your diet are:

Leafy Greens: Spinach, kale, and Swiss chard are packed with magnesium and can be easily added to salads, smoothies, or stir-fries.

- **Nuts and Seeds:** Almonds, cashews, and pumpkin seeds are great sources of magnesium, and they make a convenient snack.
- **Whole Grains:** Brown rice, quinoa, and oats are high in magnesium and provide additional fiber to support digestion.
- **Legumes:** Black beans, lentils, and kidney beans are not only high in protein but also rich in magnesium.
- **Bananas:** In addition to potassium (which we'll discuss next), bananas are a good source of magnesium, making them an excellent snack option.

Incorporating these foods into your meals will help ensure your muscles stay healthy and reduce the risk of cramping or discomfort. You can also consider magnesium supplements if needed, but it's always best to talk to a healthcare provider before adding any new supplements to your routine.

Potassium: Balancing Muscle Function and Preventing Cramps

Potassium is another key nutrient that helps regulate muscle function. It works alongside sodium to maintain fluid balance in your cells and muscles, which is critical for proper muscle contraction. When potassium levels are low, you might experience muscle weakness, cramps, or even spasms, which can interfere with physical activity and exercises aimed at improving scoliosis. Since muscles rely on potassium to contract and relax effectively, ensuring adequate intake can help improve your ability to maintain proper posture and muscle balance.

Some potassium-rich foods that can help support your muscle function include:

- **Bananas:** Perhaps the most famous potassium-rich food, bananas are a convenient and delicious way to boost your potassium intake. They're easy to incorporate into smoothies or eat as a snack.
- **Sweet Potatoes:** These are not only a great source of potassium, but also packed with fiber and vitamins, making them a nutritious option for muscle health.
- **Avocados:** Avocados are a rich source of potassium and healthy fats, which can support overall muscle health and provide energy.
- **Spinach:** This leafy green is high in both magnesium and potassium, making it a great addition to your diet for supporting muscles and bones.
- **Oranges:** A refreshing source of potassium, oranges are also packed with vitamin C, which supports collagen

production for healthy muscles and connective tissue.

Eating a balanced diet with adequate potassium will help ensure your muscles function optimally and prevent cramps or spasms during your isometric exercises. Combining potassium-rich foods with protein and magnesium can provide comprehensive muscle support for your scoliosis management.

Combining Protein, Magnesium, and Potassium for Optimal Muscle Health

For those managing scoliosis, keeping muscles strong and functioning properly is key to supporting the spine and improving posture. Protein, magnesium, and potassium work together to ensure your muscles have the building blocks, energy, and function they need to perform at their best. When you combine these nutrients in your diet, you'll be better equipped to handle the demands of isometric exercises and daily activities.

Make sure to include a variety of protein sources, magnesium-rich foods, and potassium-packed options in your meals. Consistency is key, so try to incorporate these nutrients into your diet every day. Consider consulting with a healthcare provider or nutritionist to ensure you're meeting your needs.

Strategic Suggestions

To support your muscles during scoliosis management, start by focusing on protein, magnesium, and potassium-rich foods in your diet. Aim for a well-rounded approach, ensuring that you get a balance of these nutrients throughout the day. As you begin to feel stronger and more energized, it may be helpful to track your intake and monitor how your muscles respond. If you experience persistent muscle issues or need guidance on the right supplements for you, consult a healthcare professional for personalized advice.

Importance of Hydration and Balanced Meals

When it comes to managing scoliosis, many people focus on the physical exercises and stretches that strengthen the muscles and support the spine. However, there's an often overlooked but crucial factor: proper hydration and balanced meals. What you eat and how well-hydrated you are can significantly impact how effectively your body responds to physical activity, including isometric exercises. Ensuring that you're properly hydrated and nourished helps your body recover, reduces muscle cramps, supports joint function, and contributes to overall well-being.

Hydration: The Foundation for Muscle Function and Joint Health

Water is essential for your body's overall function. In fact, about 60% of your body weight is made up of water, and it's involved in almost every bodily function, from nutrient transport to temperature regulation. When you're properly hydrated, your muscles and joints perform better. Dehydration, on the other hand, can lead to fatigue, muscle cramps, poor performance in physical activity, and increased discomfort—especially for those managing scoliosis.

Hydration helps maintain the fluid balance in your cells, ensuring that your muscles can contract and relax properly. Water also plays a crucial role in joint lubrication, reducing friction and preventing stiffness, which can be a concern for people with scoliosis who already experience uneven wear on their joints. Staying hydrated is especially important when engaging in any physical activity, including isometric exercises, because it helps your body efficiently process nutrients and remove waste products produced by your muscles.

How Much Water Should You Drink?

The amount of water you need can vary depending on factors like age, activity level, and climate. However, a general recommendation is to aim for at least eight 8-ounce glasses of water per day, known as the "8x8" rule. If you're engaging in physical activity, especially exercises that target your muscles like isometric holds, you may need more hydration to account for the fluids lost through sweat.

Here are a few tips for staying hydrated:

1. Drink Water Throughout the Day

Rather than waiting until you're thirsty, aim to sip water consistently throughout the day. Keep a water bottle with you as a reminder to drink.

Increase Intake During Exercise: If you're working out or doing isometric exercises, drink more water before, during, and after the activity to replenish fluids lost through sweat.

2. Add Electrolytes if Needed

If you're engaging in intense exercise or live in a hot climate, you may need more than just water. Adding an electrolyte drink or consuming foods high in electrolytes (like bananas, oranges, or coconut water) can help replenish minerals lost in sweat.

Proper hydration can have a positive effect on your energy levels, muscle recovery, and ability to perform isometric exercises. If you're dehydrated, you might find that your muscles feel weaker, or you're more prone to cramping. Keeping your body hydrated helps maintain your muscle health and supports your ability to maintain proper posture—an important aspect when managing scoliosis.

Balanced Meals: Fueling Your Body for Optimal Performance

While hydration is vital, what you eat is equally important when managing scoliosis and supporting your body's muscles and joints. A balanced meal provides the nutrients necessary for muscle function, bone strength, and overall health. Focus on nutrient-dense foods that are rich in vitamins, minerals, protein, and healthy fats. Eating a variety of these foods will provide your body with the fuel it needs to handle physical activities like isometric exercises and support spine health.

A balanced meal should consist of three key components:

1. Protein

Protein is essential for muscle repair and growth, especially after physical activities that involve muscle contraction. Good sources of protein include lean meats, fish, eggs, legumes, nuts, and seeds.

2. Carbohydrates

Carbohydrates are your body's main source of energy. Opt for whole grains, fruits, and vegetables to ensure you're getting complex carbs that provide sustained energy throughout the day. Avoid highly processed foods and refined sugars that can cause energy crashes.

3. Healthy Fats

Healthy fats, such as those found in avocados, olive oil, nuts, and fatty fish, are essential for reducing inflammation and supporting overall joint health. Omega-3 fatty acids, in particular, can help reduce joint pain and stiffness.

When you're planning your meals, make sure you're getting a variety of foods to ensure that you're not missing out on any essential nutrients. For example, a balanced meal could be a piece of grilled chicken (protein) with a side of quinoa (carbs) and a serving of steamed broccoli (fiber, vitamins, and minerals), drizzled with olive oil (healthy fats).

Meals for Muscle and Bone Support

When you're managing scoliosis, it's important to focus on meals that not only fuel your muscles but also support your bones. Bone-strengthening nutrients like calcium and vitamin D are essential for those with scoliosis, as they help maintain bone density and prevent the progression of the condition. Include dairy products, leafy greens, and fortified foods in your meals to ensure you're getting adequate calcium and vitamin D.

Examples of Balanced Meals for Scoliosis Support

Here are some meal ideas that provide a balanced mix of nutrients to support your muscles, bones, and overall health:

1. Breakfast

Scrambled eggs with spinach and avocado on whole-grain toast, accompanied by a glass of fortified milk or a smoothie with calcium and vitamin D.

2. Lunch

Grilled chicken salad with mixed greens, quinoa, cherry tomatoes, and olive oil dressing. Add a side of roasted sweet potatoes for extra fiber and potassium.

3. Dinner

Baked salmon with steamed broccoli, brown rice, and a side of roasted vegetables like carrots and bell peppers. This meal provides healthy fats, protein, fiber, and essential vitamins and minerals.

4. Snacks

Greek yogurt with nuts and berries, or a banana with almond butter for a protein and potassium boost.

The Role of Balanced Meals in Your Isometric Routine

Just like hydration, balanced meals are essential to your isometric exercise routine. If your body doesn't have the proper nutrients, your muscles may not recover as well, and your performance might decline. A well-rounded diet provides the energy your body needs to engage in muscle-strengthening exercises and maintain proper posture. When your body is properly fueled, you can perform exercises like wall sits, planks, and other holds with more stamina and less discomfort.

Next Steps for Better Hydration and Nutrition

To support your scoliosis management, start by focusing on staying hydrated and eating balanced, nutrient-rich meals. Ensure you're drinking enough water throughout the day and eating meals that include a mix of protein, carbohydrates, and healthy fats. Incorporating nutrient-dense foods will not only help with muscle and bone health but also contribute to your overall well-being. If you ever feel unsure about your hydration or nutrition plan, consider talking to a dietitian or healthcare provider for personalized advice.

Strategic Suggestions

Proper hydration and balanced meals are key elements in your scoliosis management. Water supports muscle function and joint health, while a nutrient-rich diet ensures that your muscles and bones receive the necessary fuel to perform well during physical activity. When you incorporate these strategies into your daily routine, you'll feel more energized, recover faster, and be better equipped to handle the demands of isometric exercises.

Chapter 10: Putting It All Together

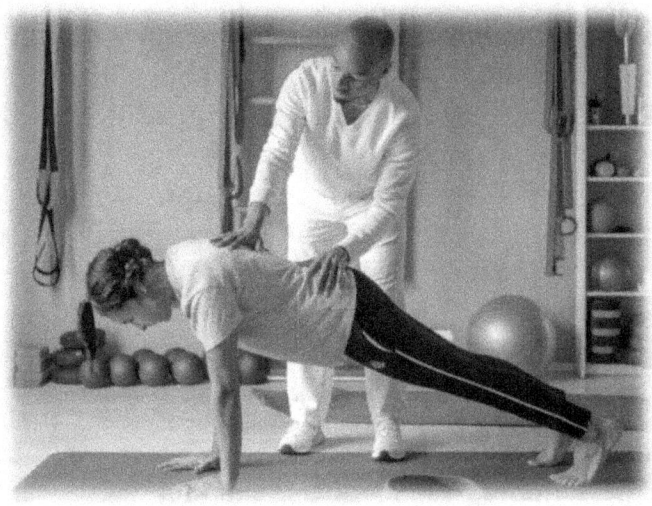

Starting a consistent exercise routine is the first step toward improving your scoliosis management. A weekly plan helps you stay on track, balancing exercise with rest while ensuring that you're targeting all the right areas of your body. This plan should not only focus on the exercises themselves but also on how you can fit them into your lifestyle for long-term success. However, with some structure and understanding of your body's needs, you'll be able to create a routine that is both effective and sustainable.

Building a Weekly Isometric Exercise Plan

Step 1: Assess Your Starting Point

Before creating your weekly plan, it's important to understand your body's current condition. Are you new to exercise, or are you familiar with isometric exercises already? Knowing your starting point will help determine how many repetitions and sets you should include. If you're just starting, begin with shorter holds and fewer repetitions. As you become more accustomed to the exercises, you can gradually increase the intensity and duration.

Also, consider any discomfort you may be experiencing. Is scoliosis causing significant pain, or is it mostly a mild issue that needs strengthening? Consult your doctor or physical therapist if necessary, as they can help you better understand your limits and guide you on how to adjust your exercises as you progress.

Step 2: Plan for a Balanced Routine

To get the most out of your isometric exercises, you'll want to ensure you're working all major muscle groups throughout the week. A well-rounded routine should incorporate core exercises, lower body work, and upper body strength, alongside exercises that specifically help posture. Here's an example of how you can structure your weekly plan:

- **Monday – Core and Upper Body Focus:** Start with exercises like planks, wall push-ups, and scapular squeezes. These will strengthen your core and upper body, focusing on the muscles that help stabilize your spine.
- **Tuesday – Lower Body Focus:** Perform wall sits, glute bridges, and modified lunges. These movements will target your legs and hips, important areas for posture control and balance.
- **Wednesday – Active Rest Day:** Take a break from intense exercises but focus on stretching and gentle movements to improve flexibility. This day can also be dedicated to mindfulness practices such as yoga or Tai Chi, which can help with spinal alignment.
- **Thursday – Core and Upper Body Focus:** Return to your plank variations and other upper body strengthening exercises to maintain muscle activation and stability.
- **Friday – Lower Body and Posture:** Include exercises such as pelvic tilts and isometric lunges. These will support both your posture and lower body strength.

- **Saturday – Active Rest Day or Light Activity:** Take another active recovery day to allow your body to rest and repair. You can go for a walk, practice light stretching, or even enjoy a swim.
- **Sunday – Full Body Review:** Do a lighter session incorporating elements from all areas of your previous exercises. This will help reinforce the balance in your routine and ensure that every muscle group is targeted.

Step 3: Gradually Increase Difficulty

When you're starting, it's important to gradually increase the intensity of your exercises. Isometric exercises are highly effective, but only if you challenge your muscles to work hard enough to improve strength. In the beginning, aim for shorter hold times—perhaps 10-15 seconds per exercise. As you get stronger, increase the duration to 30-60 seconds, depending on your comfort level.

In addition to hold time, consider increasing the number of sets or repetitions you perform. For example, start with two sets of each exercise, and work up to three or four as your body adapts. Remember that progression is key, but do not rush. Focus on quality and proper form rather than pushing for maximum reps or duration too soon.

Step 4: Listen to Your Body

One of the most important aspects of any exercise plan is paying attention to how your body feels. Isometric exercises should challenge your muscles without causing pain. If you experience discomfort or pain, stop the exercise immediately and adjust your technique or intensity. Overexertion can lead to injury, so it's essential to maintain proper form and take breaks when needed. If you're unsure about your progress or experience pain, it's always wise to seek professional advice from a physical therapist or trainer experienced in scoliosis.

Step 5: Track Your Progress

Finally, tracking your progress will help keep you motivated and show you how far you've come. You can keep a simple exercise log where you record the number of sets, hold time, and how you felt after each session. Tracking your improvements will help you feel a sense of accomplishment and encourage you to stay consistent with your weekly routine.

Strategic Suggestions

Building a weekly isometric exercise plan for scoliosis doesn't have to be complicated, but it does require consistency and patience. As you continue, remember that it's okay to adjust your plan as you go. The goal is to gradually increase strength and stability in a sustainable way. With time, you'll feel more comfortable and confident in your exercises, helping you manage your scoliosis more effectively.

Combining Isometric Workouts with Other Treatments

While isometric exercises are a powerful tool for managing scoliosis, combining them with other treatments can help you achieve better results. Each approach offers unique benefits, and when combined, they create a comprehensive strategy for supporting your spine, improving posture, and reducing pain. This section will guide you on how to combine isometric workouts with other treatments for scoliosis to create a holistic approach that works best for you.

Step 1: Physical Therapy as a Supportive Treatment

Physical therapy plays a crucial role in scoliosis management. A physical therapist can help you develop a personalized treatment plan that may include isometric exercises, but also stretches and other exercises designed to improve spinal alignment, mobility, and flexibility. They can assess your scoliosis curve and recommend modifications to certain exercises to avoid unnecessary strain on your spine. They will also help you address specific issues like muscle imbalances, which are common in people with scoliosis.

For instance, a physical therapist might guide you in performing corrective exercises that target areas such as the upper back and hips. These exercises, when combined with your isometric routine, can promote better posture and prevent the compensatory movements that often arise from scoliosis.

Step 2: Stretching and Mobility Work

In addition to strength-building exercises like isometric holds, incorporating stretching and mobility work is essential for maintaining flexibility and preventing stiffness in the spine. A stretching routine can help lengthen the muscles surrounding your spine, which can reduce discomfort and improve your range of motion.

You can combine static stretching, which involves holding a stretch for a set period, with dynamic stretching, which incorporates movement to improve flexibility. For example, adding gentle spinal twists or stretches for your hamstrings, hip flexors, and lower back can complement your isometric exercises. These stretches help to maintain a balance between flexibility and strength, which is crucial for scoliosis management.

Consider performing a 5–10 minute stretching routine before and after your isometric workouts. This can help loosen tight muscles and reduce tension in your spine. Yoga or Pilates can also be beneficial as they promote flexibility, alignment, and mindful movements.

Step 3: Ergonomic Adjustments for Better Posture

Your daily habits, such as sitting, standing, and sleeping, can have a significant impact on your scoliosis. Ergonomics refers to the science of designing the environment around you to promote better posture and comfort. Small changes in your environment can make a big difference in reducing strain on your spine and improving your posture, which ultimately supports your isometric exercises.

For example, if you work at a desk for long hours, ensure that your workstation is set up in a way that encourages good posture. Keep your computer screen at eye level, use a chair with good lumbar support, and avoid slouching or rounding your shoulders. When sitting, focus on sitting up straight with your feet flat on the floor and your knees at a 90-degree angle. You can also place a small cushion or lumbar roll in the small of your back for additional support.

At night, make sure your mattress and pillow are providing the right level of support. Sleeping on your side with a pillow between your knees or on your back with a cushion under your knees can help maintain a neutral spine alignment while you sleep.

Step 4: Medical Interventions for Severe Scoliosis

In some cases, scoliosis may require more than just exercise and physical therapy. If your scoliosis curve is moderate to severe, your doctor may recommend additional treatments such as bracing or even surgery. A scoliosis brace can help reduce the curvature of the spine by applying gentle pressure, and it is often worn during the growing years.

For more severe cases, spinal surgery may be considered. Surgery is generally reserved for individuals with curves that are progressing rapidly or causing significant pain and dysfunction. However, even if surgery is an option, combining it with post-surgical isometric exercises can help speed up recovery and improve long-term outcomes.

It's crucial to work closely with your healthcare provider to determine the best treatment plan based on your individual needs. They can guide you on how to incorporate isometric exercises into your regimen, especially if you're recovering from surgery or wearing a brace.

Step 5: Consistency and Holistic Approach

The key to success when combining isometric exercises with other treatments is consistency. Incorporating a combination of exercise, therapy, stretching, and ergonomic adjustments into your daily routine will give you the best chance for long-term scoliosis management. Remember that improvement takes time, so stay patient and consistent.

It's also important to view your treatment plan as a holistic approach to overall well-being, not just a series of exercises. You're not just focusing on your spine, but on strengthening the muscles, improving posture, and reducing discomfort in your entire body. A comprehensive plan will not only help improve your scoliosis but also contribute to your overall health.

Strategic Suggestions

Combining isometric exercises with other treatments is a powerful way to manage scoliosis. When you integrate physical therapy, stretching, ergonomic adjustments, and even medical interventions, you can create a treatment plan that supports your spine and overall health. With patience and consistency, you'll likely see improvement in both your scoliosis and quality of life.

Sustaining Long-Term Results

Once you've established a solid foundation of isometric exercises and other treatments for your scoliosis, the next challenge is sustaining those positive results over the long term. Achieving improvements in posture, strength, and flexibility is a major accomplishment, but maintaining those changes requires ongoing commitment and consistency. Sustaining long-term results from your isometric exercises and other treatments is all about consistency, lifestyle changes, and continuous self-care. As you begin to see improvements in your scoliosis management, it's important to stay focused on maintaining those gains. Your body will adapt over time, so it's essential to remain proactive about your routine, modify it as needed, and make adjustments to fit your evolving needs.

Step 1: Create a Sustainable Routine

One of the keys to sustaining long-term results is creating a workout routine that you can stick to. It's important to find a balance between challenging yourself and maintaining consistency. If your routine is too difficult, you might burn out or injure yourself; if it's too easy, you won't see continued improvement. A sustainable routine is one that you can realistically fit into your lifestyle, without feeling overwhelmed or stressed.

Start by establishing a weekly schedule for your isometric exercises. Aim for at least 3–4 sessions per week, gradually increasing the duration and intensity of the holds as you become more comfortable. Incorporate your exercises into a well-rounded fitness plan that includes stretching, aerobic activity, and strength training. You can also alternate your focus each day – for example, one day focusing on core exercises, another on lower body, and another on upper body, to keep things fresh and prevent overuse injuries.

Step 2: Progress Slowly and Gradually

As you progress in your scoliosis management, remember that slow, gradual changes are more sustainable than making drastic jumps in intensity or duration. If you push yourself too hard too quickly, you risk injury or burnout. Instead, aim for small, consistent progress. Gradually increase the length of each isometric hold by 5 to 10 seconds each week, or increase the difficulty of the exercises by slightly changing your angle or position.

Tracking your progress can help keep you motivated and encourage small wins along the way. Keep a workout journal to log your exercise sessions, noting the exercises you performed, how long you held each position, and how you felt afterward. Over time, you'll notice improvements, such as being able to hold a plank for a longer period or feeling less discomfort after your exercises.

Step 3: Listen to Your Body

Listening to your body is one of the most important aspects of sustaining long-term results. While pushing through some discomfort during isometric exercises is normal (since they target deep muscles), pain is not. If you experience sharp or intense pain, stop immediately and assess your form. Ensure that you're performing each exercise correctly and that you're not straining your spine in the process.

Take breaks when necessary and give your body time to rest. This is especially important if you experience any soreness after your workouts. Rest and recovery are just as important as the exercises themselves.

Step 4: Keep Incorporating Other Treatment Methods

As your isometric exercises become a regular part of your life, continue to incorporate other treatments into your routine. Physical therapy, stretching, ergonomic adjustments, and even medical treatments should remain a consistent part of your scoliosis management plan. These methods work together to promote a balanced and holistic approach to spinal health.

For example, if you're focusing more on isometric exercises for strength, don't forget about stretching and mobility work to keep your muscles flexible and prevent tightness. Also, if your scoliosis is mild, you may need to re-evaluate your posture regularly throughout the day, such as if you're sitting at a desk, standing, or sleeping. Small adjustments over time can have a big impact on your long-term health.

Step 5: Monitor and Adjust as Needed

Over time, your body will adapt to the exercises you're doing, and you may reach a point where you don't see as much progress. This is a natural part of the process, and when it happens, it's time to adjust your routine. This might involve increasing the intensity of your exercises, adding new variations, or focusing on different muscle groups.

Additionally, it's important to check in with your healthcare provider periodically. They can assess your progress and make adjustments to your treatment plan if needed. If you're working with a physical therapist, they can help guide you through more advanced exercises as your strength and flexibility improve.

Step 6: Focus on Lifestyle Factors

To sustain your results, it's also essential to take care of your overall health and lifestyle. Nutrition plays a significant role in muscle repair and bone health, so continue to focus on a balanced diet rich in calcium, vitamin D, protein, and magnesium. Sleep is another crucial factor in recovery, so make sure you're getting adequate rest each night to allow your body to heal and rebuild.

Staying active outside of your isometric workouts is also important. Engaging in low-impact activities like walking, swimming, or cycling can help keep your muscles strong and maintain mobility. You might also consider adding yoga or Pilates to your routine, as they help improve flexibility, balance, and alignment, which are especially beneficial for scoliosis.

Strategic Suggestions

Sustaining long-term results from your isometric exercises and scoliosis management requires consistency, gradual progression, and ongoing self-care. When you stick to a manageable routine, listen to your body, and incorporate other treatments and lifestyle factors, you can continue to see improvements and maintain a strong, healthy spine. Don't be afraid to adjust your plan as needed, and always keep an eye on your long-term health goals.

Conclusion